Breathe and Let Go

A Lung Transplant Adventure

Gavin Maitland

To Eleanor

Best wishes

Gavin Maitland

First published by Dog Ear Publishing
4010 W. 86th Street, Ste H
Indianapolis, IN 46268
www.dogearpublishing.net

dog ear PUBLISHING

ISBN: 978-160844-333-8

This book is printed on acid-free paper.

Printed in the United States of America

To Julie, Alex and Riley

PROLOGUE

It was an early spring Colorado day: cold and clear. As I launched myself into the pool at the start of the Blaster Blast triathlon on April 19th, 2009, I didn't even notice the cold. I started to swim with the slow easy front crawl style I had perfected over years. I rolled my head every second stroke, and drew in a wonderfully deep breath as I felt my lungs working harder and harder. It was an easy distance this first time, only 400 meters, and I overtook two or three other competitors who had started before me.

I felt strong as I hauled myself out of the pool at the end of the swimming stage of the event. I dashed outside, dripping wet, to the transition area where my bike stood, carefully prepared for the cycling stage. I barely dried myself. I slipped on my helmet, shoved on my running shoes, and set off on my bike at a good pace. My breathing was deep and steady.

Six laps - twelve miles - of the Colorado School of Mines' campus followed. My breathing became more and more labored as I pushed through the fatigue in my legs for the uphill sections of the course. The wind whipped across my face as I coasted on the down-hill part of the course, allowing me to catch my breath. At the end of the biking segment, I leaped off my bike, tore off my helmet and started to run. My legs wobbled a bit as they got used to the transition of the concrete surface from the smooth peddling action of the bike. My breathing was steady and smooth, as I ran on the path alongside a meandering creek. It was only a three mile run, but it felt much longer. I pushed on, running slowly but steadily.

At last, the finish line was in sight, only minutes away. Hearing the cheers of friends and other spectators, I involuntarily sped up. My friends had spread the word amongst the remaining spectators that I was a double lung transplant recipient, one of a mere handful who had ever completed a triathlon, so I received a rapturous welcome when I crossed the finish line. I slowed to a walk, and let the moment wash over me. I was tired, but not out of breath. My breathing was clear, slow, deep and steady. I had done it. Just over a year after my double lung transplant on March 14th, 2008, I had completed my first triathlon.

*****

CHAPTER 1

Waking Up

When I woke up from the lung transplant surgery, I couldn't see, I couldn't speak and I couldn't move. My hands were tied – not uncomfortably, but tied nonetheless – to the sides of the bed. I knew this was going to happen, as we had been through extensive briefings about the surgery and the hospital stay, but, at the same time, I had to resist the instinct to panic. I took a deep breath. Despite my anesthesia-induced state of drowsiness, I remember thinking, "Wow, I can breathe!"

I took another deep breath. I could feel my diaphragm expanding as my chest filled with beautiful air, and I smiled as I exhaled, lying there in the darkness.

It was a feeling I could remember, but hadn't experienced in years. The deterioration of my lungs over the past five years meant that my breathing had steadily become more and more restricted. Each breath had become short and shallow as my body struggled to get the oxygen it needed. My lung capacity had shrunk to an alarming thirty percent of what was normal for someone of my age.

But now, that felt better. I took another deep breath, relishing in the depth to which I could push my diaphragm out and the feeling of my two new lungs expanding my chest.

I was aware of people in the room with me. I knew my hands were tethered to the bedside to stop me from involuntarily reaching over and pulling out the breathing tube that was down my throat. I didn't know why I couldn't see, but for some reason, I couldn't open my eyes. I was aware that my wife, Julie, was standing next to me by the bed, and was saying something to me. I strained to listen, but couldn't make out what she was saying.

I flexed the fingers on my right hand. They felt stiff and unresponsive. I opened and closed my hand several times.

"Walk," they had said. *"It is vitally important that you walk as soon as possible after your operation, so that you can begin to use your new lungs."*

All I could hear in my head was *"Walk! You must get up and walk!"* I started to move my index and middle fingers. My fingers felt stiff, but I pushed them to squiggle into what I thought was a walking motion.

"What's he doing?" I heard my wife Julie say. "Why is he doing that?" She probably thought that I was having some kind of spasm in my hand. I could tell that she didn't understand what I was doing, so I made a gesture of holding a pen. "Give me a pen to write with!" I wanted to say, but I couldn't make a sound.

I heard Julie reacting: "Get a pen, he wants to write!" A minute later, I felt a pen in my hand and started to scrawl the word W-A-L-K on the paper that was beneath my hand.

"He wants to walk! He wants to walk!" I heard Julie shout jubilantly. She sounded very relieved.

Afterwards, Julie told me how comical the situation was. I was lying in bed in the intensive care unit of the Duke University Medical Center hospital, with what seemed to be a million tubes coming out of me, connected to all kinds of boxes, drips and electronic equipment, a twenty-four-inch scar across my chest, and a respirator in my mouth. I had just come out of a five-and-a half hour operation that had replaced both of my lungs. When Julie said "He wants to walk!" the nurse just looked at her somberly and said, "I don't think so."

******

Progress came fast – or maybe it just seemed that way as I lapsed in and out of consciousness. The doctors removed the respirator from my mouth and released my hands. I remember feeling too hot and too cold at the same time. I asked the nurse to give me bags of ice cubes, which I put under my feet. The tightness of my skin made me squirm with discomfort.

I felt strange from the effects of all of the new drugs that had been introduced in the past twelve hours, as well as the aftermath of the anesthetic. I was also experiencing the first effects of massive doses of prednisone, an anti-inflammatory and immuno-suppressive drug intended to prevent my body from rejecting my new lungs. In the weeks leading up to the transplant operation, I had been on five milligrams. During the operation, the dosage had jumped to a whopping 500 milligrams, 100 times the amount I had received earlier. No wonder I felt uncomfortable.

Are You Pedro?

One of the more unpleasant aspects of the hospital stay post-transplant is the daily ritual of a bronchoscopy for new lung recipients.

The only way pulmonologists can get an accurate picture of how the new lungs are settling in is to insert a three foot-long-tube, with a tiny camera on the end, down through the nostrils and into the depths of the lungs to take a sample of the tissue to look for abnormalities. And I wasn't going to be given much of a break. Hours after waking up from the surgery, the first of many bronchoscopies would be performed.

Jeff, one of my new friends from the rehabilitation center (the Center for Living at Duke University Medical Center), who had his transplant a few weeks prior to me, told me to expect a visit from a doctor called Pedro Catarino, who would administer the unpleasantness. Accordingly, every time anyone remotely resembling a doctor would stick his or her head into my room, I would ask with trepidation "Are you Pedro?"

It sounds ridiculous looking back at my surprise at this, but there is a guy in the intensive care unit whose job it is to keep patients clean and hygienic. He came into my room and asked me if I wanted to have my hair washed with a special washing cap that they must only use in hospitals. I readily agreed, and remember saying to him, "Yes, that's great, but are you Pedro?"

Eventually, Pedro arrived. He was a sprightly young doctor with an English accent and Portuguese ancestry. He cheerfully introduced me to the bronchoscopy unit, assuring me that it would be a little uncomfortable, but not painful. In my semi-conscious state, I just put my head back as instructed and let him get on with it. Luckily, I was still feeling the numbing effects of the anesthetic, so it wasn't too bad. I remember thinking that this was a type of discomfort that I would need to get used to in my new life.

I knew from earlier briefings that I would be kept "dry" after the transplant operation, as the doctors believed that the new lungs settled in much better in a dry environment. In practice, that meant that for several weeks after the operation I got all my nutrition through an intravenous drip, and I wasn't allowed to drink anything, not even a sip of water or a single ice cube. My mouth was parched. It was the driest sensation that I had ever experienced.

Julie had left by now, exhausted by the marathon session of anxious waiting, along with her father, Larry, who had flown in from Tucson in Arizona to be with us.

I was having longer periods of consciousness. I remember trying to focus my eyes on the on-duty nurse who was monitoring all the dials and lights in my room. A large bottle of mineral water was sitting on her desk, torturing me, and she paused and took a long drink. "Could you get rid of that bottle of water, please?" I croaked. She looked surprised, but nonetheless took the bottle out of the room.

I must have woken up again as a couple of nurses pushed an x-ray film onto the illuminated screen on the wall of the screen. They didn't know that I was conscious enough to be listening to what they were saying. "Boy, these lungs look great," one of them said.

I felt a surge of relief at their affirmation that the lungs were clear and healthy – I had actually never doubted that they would be – although I also felt uncomfortable that they were reading the x-ray right in front of me. What if the lungs weren't in good condition? Would they have said out loud, "Boy, these lungs are in terrible shape!" Happily, though, that wasn't the case for me. I drifted back to sleep.

******

Time is a strange concept when you are in a windowless hospital room and drifting in and out of consciousness. There was no clock on the wall, and I had given up my watch before the operation. I knew that I had been wheeled into the operating room at about 2:00 a.m. on Friday morning, and that the operation had begun at about 4:30 a.m. and was over by 10:00 a.m., five-and-a-half hours later, when I was moved from the operating room into the intensive care unit.

I was lapsing in and out of consciousness during the day on Friday and it wasn't until evening that I started to feel coherent again. My idea of walking didn't seem so crazy anymore. I asked the nurse again if it was time yet to get up to walk. She said not yet, but maybe soon, adding that I just needed to be patient, a commodity that I would need a lot of over the coming days, weeks and months of recovery.

Ready to Take a Walk Yet?

At about midnight on Friday night, just eighteen hours after receiving my new lungs, a fit looking man in jogging gear came into my room in the intensive care unit.

"How do you feel?" he asked in a direct way. He introduced himself as John, the physical therapist who would help get me up. "Are you ready to take a walk yet?" he asked.

"Sure thing," I replied, but what about all this stuff?" I gestured at the many drainage tubes coming from my body, as well as the drip, the blood pressure cuff, and the epidural wire that was coming from my back.

"We'll take it all with us!" John replied cheerfully. With the expertise of a practiced surgeon, he deftly piled up all my boxes and connectors onto two stands on wheels, and proudly announced "Okay, we're ready!"

I gingerly swung my legs out of bed, mindful of the catheter that I could suddenly feel. John helped me to put on some slippers, and I stood up. He was standing over me as if I was about to keel over, but I waved him away. "I feel fine," I lied. 'Let's go!"

He pushed a walker over to me, and I grasped the handles. I shuffled out of the intensive care unit and out into the corridor, feeling like I was a hundred years old. Cautiously, I moved along, walking past several other transplant patients who were in various states of consciousness in their glass-fronted rooms. Together, John and I walked down the corridor at a snail's pace, balancing all my accompanying accessories on the wheeling stands. We got to the end of the corridor, turned around, and started back to my room. "How do you feel?" John asked.

"Generally, I feel fine," I replied. And I did feel fine, considering what my body had just been through. I could walk, I could breath on my own and despite all the accessories that I was trailing around after me, one accessory was conspicuous by its absence: my portable oxygen unit. I no longer needed supplementary oxygen. I felt like punching the air with elation.

We got back to my room, and I carefully climbed back into my bed. My legs were shaking from the exertion, and probably also from the effect of the drugs.

"Well done," said John. "You'll do fine." He was beaming broadly.

Standing Ovation

A couple of hours later, around 2:00 a.m. on Saturday morning, a nurse came into my room. "We think you are ready to go to the stepdown unit. Are you okay with that?" she asked.

"Absolutely," I replied. I knew that patients weren't discharged from the intensive care unit until they were stable and ready, so I was pleased that I had progressed to the next stage.

"Do you want to walk there?" The nurse asked. "It's not very far, only 100 yards or so."

"Yes, I'll try," I said. So the nurse called a colleague, and together they loaded all my drainage boxes, the drips, and other accessories onto the wheeling stands, and helped me out of bed again. I walked as upright as I could, with as much dignity as I could muster, along the corridor towards the stepdown unit. As I passed the nurses' station at the entrance to the stepdown unit, there were three or four nurses there. The nurse accompanying me said to them, "Look at this! He's walking just twenty-four hours after his transplant!"

The nurses at the station all stood up and started applauding as I shuffled past. I think that is the only standing ovation I have ever received in my life. I managed a smile and a wave as I went by. As I reached my room, it seemed as if I had just overcome a Himalayan obstacle. I was uncomfortable, tired and spaced-out, but at the same time I was excited and relieved that I had passed the first physical test in this whole process. I was ready for whatever was next.

CHAPTER 2

A Six-Year Search For Answers

I have always enjoyed athletics, more as a participant than a spectator. From my point of view, the more demanding the physical challenge, the better; hence my determination to compete in the April 2009 triathlon in Golden, Colorado. It goes almost without saying that I have never smoked, have generally eaten well and followed a healthy lifestyle all my life.

All through school, while I attended Fraserburgh Academy in Aberdeenshire, Scotland, I swam in the local swimming club, rising at 7:00 a.m. five mornings a week to train before school, as well as on Saturdays. Later, at Gordonstoun School in Morayshire, Scotland, I held the school record for the 100-meter freestyle distance, despite being on a more restricted training regimen. As the school timetable only made allowance to swim twice a week at Gordonstoun, I used to surreptitiously jog back to my boarding house from rugby practice in the afternoons, pick up my swim suit and towel, and jog a mile or so over to the swimming pool. The pool was locked and unused at that time in the afternoons, so I would go up to the unlocked spectators' gallery and drop down in the semi-darkness to the pool-side. That way, I could get in another two or three clandestine swimming workouts per week.

At university in the Scottish city of Dundee, I competed on the swimming team against other Scottish universities for four years and competed every year at the annual Scottish Universities' Championship. My best strokes were freestyle and butterfly. I enjoyed competing, but more than anything, I loved feeling fit and strong. There is no finer sensation than the feeling of air rushing through your lungs as you swim hard and fast, drawing breath in and out as you go churning through the water. It is a sense of exhilaration that has no equal.

As I moved through my twenties and into my thirties, I had less time to find convenient swimming pools and turned my attention to long-distance running. I must have competed in fifty or more half-marathons, 20ks, 10ks, and other running events over the years. Among the many highlights were completing all twenty-six miles, 385 yards of the London Marathon in the two consecutive years of 1998 and 1999, as well as the New York City Marathon in 2000.

I remember feeling very disappointed with my finishing time at the New York City Marathon. The two occasions I had competed in the London Marathon, I had finished in around four hours, but I finished the New York City marathon in just under five hours. I felt that something wasn't quite right with me, but I couldn't put my finger on what it was. It would be difficult to try to explain to a doctor that I was concerned because my marathon time was a little slow. Who would be sympathetic to that?

Julie and I met in Amsterdam in 1996, where we were both working, and got married in 1998 in Aspen, Colorado. We had been contemplating a move for some time, and were not exactly sure where we would call home. Julie is an American citizen and had grown up in Colorado, so she was familiar with the area. We decided that the outdoors, space and sunshine of Colorado would be a good environment for us and our two children, Alex, then three years old and Riley, then one year old. Being a British citizen, I needed a permanent resident card for the United States, so I applied late in 2001, and got the required permission by December. In March of 2002, we moved from London to Denver, Colorado. We settled in well in Colorado, with its easy blend of friendly people and temperate climate – even in the winter. I kept exercising as normal, jogging most mornings along one of the many biking paths around our apartment building.

Around the end of 2002, I noticed that I had a persistent and irritating cough that would not go away. It is difficult to pinpoint exactly when it started, as I thought it was the symptoms of a lingering cold, but it was always there, worse when I went jogging and got out of breath.

Periodically, I would go and see a doctor, and explain my symptoms. On taking my medical history – i.e. a history of good health, no bad habits, such as smoking, no family history of respiratory problems and no obvious environmental exposure issues – the doctors would invariably declare that I must have some kind of allergy or asthma that was making me cough. The explanation always seemed to be inadequate, as I had never had any kind of allergies before, never had any symptoms of asthma, and the dry cough persisted day and night, summer and winter. But the symptoms seemed scarcely to warrant concern that a major underlying lung disease was lurking in my chest.

By January 2004, my cough had become a constant irritation. It was difficult to carry on a conversation, a phone call or a business meeting with the incessant coughing. Although it was irritating for me, it was doubly so for Julie and for other people with whom I came into contact. I decided to go and see the top specialist I could find to get the issue rooted out once and for all. I made an appointment to see a pulmonologist at National Jewish Health, which was located right in Denver, where I lived.

National Jewish Health is listed as the top respiratory hospital in the United States by the magazine *US News and World Report*. It had been located in Denver since its founding in 1899, when people believed – erroneously, as it turned out – that the dry air and constant sunshine of the Denver climate was beneficial for nasty lung diseases such as tuberculosis.

So, secure in the knowledge that National Jewish Health was the best of the best, the top of the heap, I confidently turned up for my appointment on a bright Friday morning, expecting a simple solution to my problem of a dry cough.

The pulmonologist went through a detailed medical history with me – my overall health, my parents' and brothers' health, any environmental exposure I may have had, and any smoking history. Everything was negative. I could see the doctor literally scratching his head in frustration.

At the end of the consultation, he concluded that I must have some kind of nasal drip irritation that was causing the cough, as he apparently couldn't think of anything else. I remember saying to him that a cough was symptomatic of an underlying condition, and was not a condition in itself. He agreed with me, but could not shed any light on why I was still coughing. I left with a prescription for a nasal rinse to use morning and night and a feeling of relief that it was not something serious.

Major League Pneumonia

Two days after my appointment at National Jewish Health, I began to feel terrible. I had flu-like symptoms of being hot and cold, with sore muscles, a temperature and a horrific cough. I could not leave my bed and lay in discomfort all weekend and into the next week. By Tuesday morning, I began coughing up rust-colored sputum, which Julie quickly realized was not a good sign. She bundled me into the car and drove me to the neighborhood hospital.

I haven't had much experience with emergency rooms. I broke my collar bone when I was fifteen years old, and remember sitting waiting for medical attention for a couple of hours before being seen, so I resigned myself to a long wait. But this was different. As I presented myself at the front desk of the ER, the receptionist asked me what was wrong. I said that I was having some trouble breathing and felt terrible. She quickly slipped an oxygen saturation meter onto my index finger to measure the amount of oxygen in my bloodstream, and looked at the reading. Her eyes widened and she brusquely reached for the telephone. Moments later an orderly appeared with a wheel chair and asked me to sit down. I was wheeled straight through to a treatment room. Given the stories of people waiting around for hours for attention at ERs, I realized that being seen so quickly was not a particularly good sign.

It turned out that I had pneumonia. I was very surprised. Pneumonia? Surely that was a condition for older people, not for a young and healthy person like me. Although I was worried by the diagnosis, I also felt relief, as I realized that this may be the underlying reason for my cough. I was admitted to the hospital and put on a powerful course of antibiotics administered by intravenous drip.

I was inundated by the same round of medical questions that I had answered innumerable times before: what was my medical history; what was my family medical history; did I have any potentially harmful environmental exposure; did I keep birds? All my answers were no, no, and no again. I could not help them with any good reasons why I had contracted this pneumonia. It took me a while to kick the infection, which required a full week in the hospital, my first use of oxygen and two consecutive rounds of antibiotics.

The doctor told Julie that that I had had a "major league" pneumonia, and that if I was an older person, my recovery would have been serious doubt. However, my young age and relatively good overall health played in my favor. I stayed in the hospital for six days, on oxygen, until my oxygen saturation levels rose above the target level of ninety percent.

My diagnosis on discharge from the hospital was Community Acquired Pneumococcal Pneumonia, which meant that the doctors assumed that I had caught the infection "somewhere out there" and that my symptoms pointed towards it being the pneumococcal strain of the infection. Due to the infectious nature of the pneumonia, I had been separated from my family while in the hospital, which I found stressful. But on Julie's suggestion, I took a flight the day after my discharge down to Tucson, Arizona, where I stayed with my father-in-law, Larry, for a further ten days to help my recovery.

CHAPTER 3

Searching for Clues

I was very weak from the bout of pneumonia, but I felt relieved that it seemed to have been treated successfully and that the doctors had written on my discharge form that I was expected to make a "full recovery." I relaxed in the Tucson winter sunshine, confident in the belief that the worst was over, certain that this was the culmination of the tiresome coughing, and that I would soon be back to my normal life.

But it was not to be: my cough had still not subsided. I kept thinking that it was a remnant from the pneumonia, but as the weeks passed, and the cough stayed, I began to think that it was something more than had been diagnosed so far. By July, I decided to give National Jewish Health another try to see if the physicians there could shed any light on my condition. Generally, I felt fine, but I was exercising less due to the cough's irritating effects.

Julie, who has a background in medicine and pharmaceuticals, did some internet research and called some of the respiratory physicians whom she knew personally. She came up with the name of the president of the American Lung Association, a pulmonologist based in Worcester, Massachusetts. She spoke to him and asked him to recommend the top specialist in the country for cough. The physician named Richard Martin, a pulmonologist based at – where else – National Jewish Health in Denver.

We made an appointment with Dr. Martin, and again, I turned up at the pulmonary clinic, confident that the country's pre-eminent pulmonologist would easily put his finger on the root of the problem. Dr. Martin was a confident, no-jokes sort of guy. He had already reviewed my medical notes so didn't waste any time with the same old questions that I had answered a million times. He looked at me with piercing eyes.

"Let's get a CT (computed tomography) scan," he said simply. The consultation lasted less than five minutes.

Two weeks later I was back in front of him, having had the CT scan the week before. I could see something was bothering him. He didn't have the same confident air that he had had two weeks before. He looked at me with his dark eyes. "There's something on your CT scan. I'm not sure what it is, but it's unusual."

"What do you mean, unusual?" I asked, with increasing trepidation.

"Well, it's just unusual," he said. "I'm perplexed."

'How can you be perplexed?" I said incredulously, "You are the top guy, the expert in this area. How can you be perplexed?"

"I just am," he said, with a shrug. "I am recommending that you get a biopsy of the right side of your lungs. Both sides are diseased, but the right side is worse. I can arrange it in the next ten days, if you like."

If I like? What choice did I have? This was worse than I had imagined. I felt terrified. A biopsy? I scarcely knew what that meant, never mind being scheduled for one.

"The biopsy itself is nothing to worry about," he said. He explained that the surgeon would make a small incision in my chest through my ribs to extract a sample from the diseased lung for further analysis. The hole in the lung would close by itself quickly after the procedure.

"You will be in hospital for one night, maybe two, after the procedure. You will be uncomfortable for about four weeks afterwards."

I left Dr. Martin's office in a daze. What the hell was wrong with me? I couldn't think straight as I made my way to my car, going back over and over what Dr. Martin had just told me. None of it made any sense.

A quick Google search at home told me that a biopsy was "a medical test involving the removal of cells or tissues from a living subject for examination to determine the presence or extent of a disease." That sounded serious. I could feel nervousness running up and down my spine as I read. After discussing it with Julie, I decided to go ahead as soon as possible. If there was bad news, I wanted to know what it was as soon as I could. I called the doctor's office and asked to be scheduled for the biopsy.

The biopsy was scheduled at the University of Colorado Hospital in Denver for two weeks later, the day before my thirty-eighth birthday.

It was recommended that Julie and I meet with the surgeon who was going to be performing the biopsy in advance of the procedure, so we set up an appointment with Dr. Mitchell. As we were waiting for him, his associate came into our room and said, "Dr. Mitchell will be with you in a moment. By the way, I've seen your CT scan. It doesn't look good!" With that, he ducked out of the room.

I couldn't believe his bluntness. Doesn't look good? What did that mean? Did that mean I was going to die or what? Julie was sitting beside me, and she burst into tears.

Dr. Mitchell was more circumspect. He showed us the CT scan. I had the vague knowledge that a chest x-ray should be black. Black was good, as it showed healthy lung tissue. I can still remember seeing the CT scan that looked like a starry sky: there were a lot of white asteroid-like dots over the black background. Not so good.

Dr. Mitchell went through the procedure that he was going to perform – a procedure called Video Assisted Thoracic Surgery, or VATS – and reassured us that it was a relatively simple one. Even so, as Julie and I left the hospital, I had an aching sensation in the pit of my stomach, but we tried to stay upbeat, believing that a positive attitude and diligence would provide a simple solution to all the issues.

The biopsy day came and went. The pain killers kept me comfortable, and the drainage tube that came out of the right side on my lower back was draining a red colored liquid. The first day and the second day passed. I was ready to be discharged, as Julie was holding the fort at home on her own, working as well as keeping our two active children busy.

Each morning, one of the doctors would burst unannounced into my room at 6:00 a.m. and look at the drainage box. He would give it a prod, then shake his head. "There's still output. Maybe one more day."

One more day passed. Then another, then another. I was getting more and more impatient. Why wouldn't they let me go home? Why wouldn't the wound in my side stop bleeding?

I had been expecting a hospital stay of one or two nights, but I spent ten nights in hospital until the doctors were satisfied that my condition was stable.

A Forty-One-Letter Rarity

A week after the biopsy, I telephoned Dr. Martin from my hospital room to ask for the results. It had crossed my mind that I had some kind of cancer, but I really did not believe that that was the case. Dr. Martin was busy, but he called me back within ten minutes.

"Well, we know what is wrong with you," he said. 'It's quite rare."

"What is it?" I asked, understandably anxious.

"Well, it's a condition called idiopathic pleuroparenchymal fibroelastosis. Or IPPFE for short," he added helpfully.

"Idio-what?" I said, feeling like I was swimming out of my depth in the waves of medical terminology.

"It's idiopathic," he said. "That just means we don't know where it comes from. Your condition is a form of pulmonary fibrosis, which means the lung tissue is hardening and becoming useless. That is why you are having a hard time breathing, and probably why you are coughing.

"What can you do about it?"

Dr. Martin paused, before sidestepping the question. "I'm going to refer you to the real expert in this area, Dr. Kevin Brown. He runs the interstitial lung disease program here at National Jewish. You'll be in good hands."

As he rung off, I sank back in my hospital chair and tried to absorb the news. I didn't have a medical background, so I found the terminology difficult to take in. But the bottom line was not good. I had some kind of degenerative lung disease that was not going to be easy to get past. The antibiotics that I had previously thought would clear things up were not going to do the trick.

The medical diagnosis seemed almost surreal. I looked at the name of the disease I had been diagnosed with – I had scribbled it down while Dr. Martin spelled it out. It was forty-one letters long. That seemed incredible to me. How could I be suffering from some ultra-rare condition with such a ridiculously long name? It felt like I was in a dream, a really bad dream. Julie told me later that, after I called her, she went straight to the computer and looked up the diagnosis. The results made her collapse onto the floor, sobbing and crying.

At least the diagnosis explained why the right side of my chest was still bleeding. As I understood it, the biopsy had gone into the most diseased area of my right lung to get a sample of the tissue for analysis. As the lung tissue was hardening in both lungs, but more so in the right lung, the tissue had a difficult job in repairing itself after the invasive biopsy, so the lung kept bleeding long after the doctors expected it to heal.

After ten days, I was discharged from the hospital and went home. Again, I hoped that the worst was behind me and I could get back to some form of normalcy. My appointment with Dr. Kevin Brown, the expert in interstitial lung disease, was scheduled for a few weeks later and I was hopeful that he would provide some answers for me at long last. Meanwhile, while I was recovering at home, my two children were an amazing source of comfort and positive energy. They did not let me dwell on my condition, but demanded attention to play games like Monopoly and Clue. Alex began taking an interest in our chess board that we left out, and he was soon confidently setting up the board and learning all the moves.

Several weeks later, I met with Dr. Brown. I had come to the conclusion that this institution was not the place for jokes or lightheartedness. Dr. Brown did not disappoint me. He was a severe looking professor type, with a beard and stern demeanor. With the expected efficiency, he had already reviewed my records, so went straight to the point, solemnly informing us that there weren't many treatment options for what I had.

The best we could do, he added, was to keep an eye on it and hope that the condition did not deteriorate any further. He did not recommend any further therapy or medications, so Julie and I left the appointment feeling dejected. But we hoped that at least there was a chance that the mysterious condition would clear itself up on its own. It was October of 2004.

CHAPTER 4

Still Searching

Several months passed after my consultation at the Interstitial Lung Disease clinic at National Jewish Health. As 2004 gave way to 2005, which gave way to 2006, I still had the persistent cough, but I generally convinced myself that I felt fine. Tellingly, however, I was exercising less and less, restricting myself to walks with our black Labrador Joe around the leafy Denver neighborhood where we lived.

I knew that the pulmonologists at National Jewish Health did not have a specific course of therapy for me, so I decided to try out some alternative solutions. I had voraciously read Dr. Andrew Weil's book "Spontaneous Healing" when I was in the hospital with pneumonia in 2004, and he seemed to have a lot of success with various alternatives to the conventional approach to illness taken by practitioners of allopathic medicine. I was intrigued by apparent solutions offered by Chinese medicine to many health issues, in particular acupuncture and herbal remedies.

I eagerly trawled the internet and came up with several acupuncture practices, Chinese herbal medicine clinics, practices that specialized in Indian ayurvedic medicine, homeopathic practitioners, reflexologists and bio-feedback specialists, as well as several alternative medicine practices that were recommended by family and friends.

Over the following twelve months or so, I tried them all, many more than once. I figured that if there was a gap in the medicine practiced by conventional doctors, then maybe that gap could be filled by the alternative practitioners. I clung to the idea that, given the right conditions, my body would heal itself.

In one instance, I consulted a psychic healer who was recommended by my yoga teacher (yes, I even took up Bikram yoga – the "hot" one – to see if it could clear the blockages in my lungs). This psychic invited me to his home on a remote hillside, where he kept a huge assortment of impressive looking devices, massage tables, books and oriental-looking designs and pictures. He took a sample of my blood, did some suction "cupping" on my back, performed a strange "ionizing" cleansing process on my feet to remove "toxins" and generally performed a variety of psychic exercises to pull me back to health. After four hours and a fee of $500, I didn't feel much different, but kept an open mind about his healing abilities. I actually went back to see him a few weeks later for the same hodgepodge of treatments, all with no results. With hindsight, the experience was quite funny, and I can see that the guy was not only not a psychic, but was absolutely nuts.

In another instance, I read about the special healing potential of mushrooms, especially a mushroom called reishi. I bought a book encouragingly entitled "Medicinal Mushrooms", which detailed how Western medicine developed penicillin, the single most valuable medicine of the twentieth century, from a fungus, which in turn spawned the entire class of life-saving antibiotics. It went on to say that there are over 100,000 species within the broad category of fungi, of which the penicillin mold is just one, and there are over 38,000 species of mushrooms. "Imagine the hidden healing potential in mushrooms, which thrive on decay and degeneration," I thought hopefully.

Based on purported studies, mainly done in China, the author strongly recommended the use of the reishi mushroom, claiming that they have special effects on the lungs. They even cited instances where they had significantly helped individuals suffering from lung diseases like bronchial asthma. Accordingly, in addition to buying reishi capsules from the local health food store, and gulping down copious quantities, I contacted a specialty store in Chinatown in San Francisco, and had a large bag of dried reishi mushrooms shipped to me. I endured several weeks of slurping down large mugs of reishi tea in the hope that they would help my deteriorating lungs to recover. After several weeks, with my family begging me to cease with the malodorous drinks, I gave up on the mushroom theory.

Juicing was my next strategy. Bookstores abound with books about the health benefits of drinking the juice fresh organic fruit and vegetables. I took the advice literally and could be found every morning in the kitchen whizzing up various concoctions. My family would tease me about my orange lips from gulping down carrot juice, as well as various other more exotic mixtures. Sadly, I can't say that I felt any different.

There is certainly no shortage of anecdotal evidence that there is a significant amount of merit in the alternative approaches. On a friend's recommendation, I found a holistic general practitioner who was a DO (Doctor of Osteopathic Medicine), who had been partly trained by Andrew Weil, MD, in an approach termed integrative medicine. Through my own research, I found out that DOs are trained in much in the same way as regular Medical Doctors, but with the addition of osteopathic manipulative medicine techniques. That sounded good and holistic to me!

Unfortunately, she focused on the fact that my breathing difficulties and weight loss were a result of either a poor diet (not true), or that it was all in my head (also not true); she believed that I was somehow creating my health problems through my own thoughts. I was less than convinced, but I followed her advice for a time, although I was sure that the issue was physiological rather than psychological.

Another suggestion she came up with was to replace my silver amalgam fillings with white composite ones. She thought that it was possible that the silver amalgam fillings may be leaking mercury into my body, with the resulting toxicity causing my lung problems. While there is some evidence that white composite fillings are not as potentially harmful as amalgam ones, there is virtually no evidence that there is any health benefit from replacing them. Indeed, many dentists consider that the risks of toxic leakage from actually drilling out the original amalgam fillings are much greater than leaving them alone. After confirming my internet research with a dentist friend, I rejected the idea of a wholesale reorganization of my mouth, and after four of these "alternative therapy" sessions, I left feeling dejected and didn't consult her again.

By 2006, I was noticeably losing weight. I had never had a weight issue and kept my body at a consistent 170 to 175 pounds all my adult life. Now my weight had dwindled to around 160 pounds. I found that it was harder and harder to maintain a regular eating schedule, partly because I restricted myself from eating certain foods that contained gluten (yes, at one point I even believed that I could have an intolerance to wheat and gluten, the protein in wheat, a condition known as celiac disease), and partly due to the fact that I was just not hungry.

After I had exhausted my fourth acupuncturist, a kindly Chinese doctor who could barely speak English (which, in my mind, added to his authenticity), and countless Chinese herbalists, chiropractors, dieticians, holistic doctors and faith healers, I felt a little despondent. I was not feeling much better, and I was still losing weight, which had now slipped to 130 pounds. My usual clothes became baggy and ill-fitting while my waist size had shrunk from a usual thirty-four inches to thirty inches. In a society that is more commonly obsessed with fighting obesity, I felt like I was the only person in America who had the problem of trying to gain weight.

Not surprisingly, I had reached a point where I didn't know what to do. I felt that I had exhausted the conventional medicine route and that I was close to exhausting any options that the world of alternative medicine had to offer. I was still losing weight and was at the point of avoiding people I knew, as they invariably commented on my gaunt and emaciated look. In public, I tried to smile and shrug it off; in private, I was tired and miserable.

It may sound strange, but when you are not in full health, you and your family make unconscious adjustments to your lifestyle to accommodate your condition. We virtually cut out all trips up to the mountains, where we used to really enjoy walking and hiking, and replaced them with slow walks to the local park near our home. There was a gradual "creep" of doing fewer and fewer physical activities rather than one significant event that showed how ill I was.

Indeed, by the summer of 2007, I knew that I was in trouble, but tried to keep a brave face on things so as not to distress Julie and Alex and Riley. We went on a road trip one long weekend in August to the town of Durango in the south-west of Colorado. The area north of Durango stands at about 8,000 feet above sea level, higher even than Denver which, as the mile-high city, stands at 5,280 feet above sea level. In Denver, there is seventeen percent less oxygen than there is at sea-level, so there is even less in Durango. I could tell as soon as we got there that I was having difficulty breathing, even with normal activity.

The reduction of oxygen in the air as a result of the extra 3,000 feet made a big difference. Julie and the kids did not even notice any effect of a change in altitude, but I certainly did. The other effect that I felt was that I completely lost my appetite while we were there. I have since learned that if one's body is starved of oxygen, then it diverts all its energy to getting as much oxygen as it can, and won't waste its precious resources on less immediately important areas, such as eating. I was relieved when we left Durango and returned to Denver.

The next two months were difficult for me. My lungs were deteriorating fast, and I found it harder and harder to breathe. Even simple tasks like walking to the mailbox at the end of our short driveway would leave me out of breath. Walking any distance with the dog was out of the question.

I Need To Go To Hospital – Right Now!

Then it happened. I couldn't take it any more. Julie and I had just returned to Denver from a three-day business trip to New Jersey on the East Coast. I found that whenever I went somewhere at sea level, I felt better – hardly surprising, as it was lack of oxygen that was contributing to my sensation of feeling so unwell.

It was Saturday morning, October 6th, 2007, and I had just got up. We didn't have any plans, just to have a leisurely day at home with Alex and Riley. I remember sinking down into a chair in our library and saying to Julie that I didn't feel well. Julie suggested that we go out for breakfast, and that maybe I would feel better. I agreed, and let her drive. Once we got the bagel place, I could barely touch my breakfast. My head sank onto the table. I was literally gasping for breath. I felt like I was suffocating. I said to Julie, "I need to go the hospital. Right now."

Julie knew that I was not kidding. She bundled me out of the restaurant and into the car and we drove to the University of Colorado Hospital, where I had had the lung biopsy performed three years before.

As when I presented myself at the ER with pneumonia back in January 2004, the receptionist measured my oxygen saturation on my index finger and I was escorted straight through the waiting room and into a treatment room.

The doctors immediately put me on supplemental oxygen, took me through to radiology where they took a chest x-ray, and asked me the list of familiar questions about health history, family history and environmental exposure. They could see from my medical records that I had had a lung biopsy at the hospital previously, so they started to review them diligently.

Several different doctors came in and out of my room, and they all asked the same type of questions. They were relieved to see that my oxygen saturation level had risen from the low eighties into the high nineties with the supplemental oxygen that I was absorbing through a cannula in my nose.

I suddenly found that I was extremely hungry. Julie went out and found a sandwich for me, and I devoured it in a couple of bites. I was surprised as I had not been hungry for the last several months. The doctor next to me smiled and explained that it must be the effect of the oxygen that had triggered my appetite. In my oxygen-starved state before, my body was focusing on breathing, not eating. Now that I had enough oxygen, my body was suddenly very hungry.

I was taken from the ER up to the main hospital and admitted to the pulmonary unit. I felt much better now that I had the supplemental oxygen, but I was becoming very worried as well. What did it mean to have supplemental oxygen? Would it repair my damaged lungs? How long would I have to stay on oxygen?

Not one of the young doctors who came in and out of my room seemed able or willing to answer any of my questions. They still seemed to be gathering information before they would make any assessments. One of the tests was to be weighed. I was surprised to see that my weight had fallen to 125 pounds, the lowest I had even been in my adult life. If my regular weight was 175 pounds that meant that I had lost almost a third of my body weight. As I sat there in my hospital gown, I could tell that I was really skinny. It was not a pleasant realization.

Time passed. Julie left to go and pick up Alex and Riley, who she had left with some friends. She did not like the idea of risking their health by taking them to the hospital. I lay on the hospital bed and contemplated my situation. I was relieved to be feeling better, but alarmed by the obvious weakness of my lungs. The next day, Sunday,

I sat and read in my hospital room for the whole day. Doctors came in periodically, and nurses breezed through every hour or so to take my vitals, like blood pressure and oxygen saturation levels and to make sure I was okay. I spent another restless night, trying to get used to the oxygen tube that was inserted into my nose and suspended around my ears.

On Monday, Julie came back to see me. We knew that the doctors were going to tell us what they thought the medical issues were. Around mid-morning, three young doctors came into my room, introducing themselves as "pulmonologists or lung doctors". The leader, a young, shaven-headed man called Dr. Linderman summarized the findings: my lungs were in bad shape, my breathing was impaired, and I was going to have to use the supplemental oxygen for some time.

"What do you mean by 'some time'?" I asked cautiously.

"Well, you are a chronic case. That means that you will need to use the oxygen for as long as you need it."

"You mean, forever?"

He had trouble looking me in the eye. He just nodded. "So we think the next step…" Linderman paused and looked away from me. He seemed nervous about what he was about to say.

"The next step…" he continued, "…is to talk to the transplant people."

I was speechless. "You mean lung transplant?" was what I wanted to say, but I couldn't get any sound out of my mouth. My mouth just opened and closed like a goldfish. I looked at Julie. Her eyes had filled with tears.

This was the first time I had ever thought about the possibility of a lung transplant. So many questions flooded through my mind I didn't know where to start. How, where, when, why…? I felt the chill of fear on my spine and my stomach churned.

Linderman seemed anxious to wind up the meeting.

"We can do it here; we have a great transplant team", he said. "I will set you up with an appointment for an initial evaluation in the next couple of weeks. They will be able to answer all your questions then, better than I can. There is no reason you need to stay here in the meantime. You can go home today if you like. We will arrange oxygen supplies for you"

He and his two colleagues left the room. Not for the first time, I fought to control my feelings of panic and confusion as Julie and I packed up my things, transferred my cannula to the portable oxygen tank, and headed home.

CHAPTER 5

"Just The Two Lungs?"

October and November of 2007 passed interminably slowly as I waited to take the first steps towards becoming a candidate for a lung transplant. I was at home, on oxygen twenty-four hours a day. After I was discharged from the University of Colorado Hospital, an oxygen company truck pulled up outside my house and the driver started to unload tank after tank of oxygen that were stored in the garage. Seeing the oxygen tanks made me very scared, as I knew that it meant that I was dependent on oxygen, and I didn't know when I would be able to escape, if ever, from my predicament. The oxygen was literally keeping me alive.

I did a lot of reading, as I could not go very far while tethered to the oxygen tank. The oxygen company had provided a unit called a concentrator that blew out oxygen, and it hummed quite loudly as it sat in the center of the main floor of our house. It was irritating, but an irritation that I had no choice but to endure. Its humming was a constant reminder that I could not breathe on my own and it marked a new stage in the deterioration of my lungs.

"All I Need Is The Air That I Breathe…"

We refer to our breath and the air we breathe all the time. As the Hollies famously crooned: *"All I need is the air that I breathe..."* Indeed, it is only when you cannot breathe that you really appreciate the wondrous work that your body does to keep you oxygenated.

The average adult at rest inhales and exhales seven or eight liters of air per minute; 11,000 liters in a day. The air that is inhaled is about twenty percent oxygen, and the air that is exhaled is about fifteen percent oxygen. That means that about five percent of the volume of air is consumed in each breath and converted to carbon dioxide.

On inhalation, we get oxygen-rich air flowing though our lungs and on into our bloodstream. As we exhale, we release carbon dioxide-heavy air back into the atmosphere. Shallow breathing is bad for us, as it limits the amount of carbon dioxide that our bodies can release. Without adequate oxygen, our bodies are more at risk from strokes, heart attacks and certain forms of cancer.

Breathing to some is as old as life itself, as when God breathed life into Adam. Genesis 2:7 tells us: "*The Lord God formed the man from the dust on the ground and breathed into his nostrils the breath of life, and the man became a living being.*"

In many languages, the words for spirit and breath are the same; Greek *pneuma*; Hebrew, *ruach*; Latin, *spiritus*, so there is an inherent connection between breath and life. In many cultures, life is believed to begin with the first breath and to end with the last breath. It is believed that it is not until the breath cycle begins that the body and spirit are connected. In fact the title I have chosen for my book: Breathe and Let Go, is a reference to the emphasis of breathing in disciplines like Yoga and Buddhism, where breath plays an important role in meditation, relaxation, and reaching higher states of consciousness.

Indeed, the English language is replete with figurative expressions into which the notion of breathing is incorporated to express a range of emotional states. When you are scared, you often say that you "lose your breath" or in trepidation you "hold your breath." It seems contradictory, as you would think that in those situations, you would want to breathe to calm your body down. If you are anxious or angry, how many times has someone said to you to 'take a deep breath and count to ten?" The word 'inspired' comes from the Latin "to breathe in" and nowadays, with the gift of breath that my lung transplant has afforded me, I frequently find myself inspired by the "breathtaking" vistas of Colorado's Rocky Mountains.

Home life continued all around me, but it was tentative as everyone was aware of my predicament. To pass the time, I read, spoke to friends on the phone and read some more.

I spoke to my friend Elaine one day. If you have the good fortune to know her, Elaine is one the nicest and most genuine people in the world. I met her in the first few days at Dundee University some twenty-two years earlier. Elaine always demonstrated a rare ability to sum up a situation in her own unique way. While we talked about what is going on, with her inimitable openness and Edinburgh lilt she asked, "So is it just two lungs then, Gavin?"

Okay, that's normally too good to pass up. As my old self, I might have made some smarty-pants comment like, "Well, I thought about also asking them to dig out that in-grown toe-nail at the same time!" or "Now would be a good time to remove that appendix and those tonsils while they're at it!" or "Just the two lungs, are you kidding me!!!"

But I didn't. I just said, "Yes. It's just the two lungs." And I thought about it. Not such a big thing really. Considering the alternative, it could be a lot worse. Just the two lungs. Not the heart. Not the brain. Not the liver nor the kidneys nor the stomach. Nor anything else. Just the two lungs. Not a bad perspective on the whole thing, really.

I had been sitting at home for six weeks by now, connected to a fifty foot tube that blew a stream of oxygen up my nose. It didn't seem like much, but two liters of oxygen per minute can feel really good when you can't breathe on your own.

I had put on twenty-five pounds of weight since I started getting enough oxygen, as well as the weight-gaining prescription drug, prednisone, up from a low of 125 pounds. My normal weight is 175 pounds, so I still couldn't consider myself back to my regular weight, but it was much better. My jeans size had dropped by four inches, so I was pleased to have regained two of the lost inches. I found that I could sit on the hard wooden bench in our kitchen again, which had been uncomfortable when I was very thin, due to the lack of natural padding on my butt.

Getting the Facts

After the referral from Dr. Linderman, we had to wait for an appointment with one of the specialized lung transplant pulmonologists to discuss next steps. Because of the wait and the enforced inactivity of my condition, I spent a lot of time contemplating my situation and trying to come to terms with the prospect of having a lung transplant. I had read that it was not uncommon for patients to perish while waiting for an organ transplant; this obviously made me very nervous and scared and I tried not to think about it. It seemed clear that I was a candidate for a lung transplant. I didn't see why I wouldn't be accepted, as I felt fit and normal apart from the condition of my lungs.

******

Just before the Thanksgiving holiday of 2007, Julie and I had an appointment at the Lung Transplant Clinic at the University of Colorado Hospital in Denver. I was really anticipating this meeting, as it would answer a lot of questions that had been building up in me.

At the appointment, we met with a confident young Asian doctor – one of the "transplant team" (other lung doctors talked about them with a certain hushed reverence in the same way as I imagine regular soldiers talk about the Special Forces). His name was Doctor Lyu.

Lyu was ready to answer a lot of our basic questions, such as, "So how do you actually get the lungs out of there?" (I had always thought that my rib cage was specifically designed to make sure the lungs do not come out very easily) and "How long would it take?" and "Would I get a general anesthetic?" and, of course, "One lung or two?" Basic questions like that.

He answered with breezy phrases like: "We just pop up the hood and change them over," while making a slicing gesture with his hand across his chest.

"It takes eight to ten hours," he added, nodding enthusiastically.

"An anesthetic?"

"Eh, yes."

"One lung or two?

"Could be either. In your case, probably two."

There was also the six hour thing. "When it happens, we will need to move quickly," said Lyu. There is only about a six hour window between obtaining donor organs and getting them into a recipient's body. As many donors are victims of motor vehicle accidents, stroke and heart attack victims, it means getting the lungs out of the deceased person, dispatching two surgeons from the lung transplant team to pick them up and delivering them safely to the hospital and the recipient. If they have to be flown, they have to be flown. All within six hours.

"We have done it in nine hours, but that is really the upper limit. We prefer to do it within six," he said.

"It's a little like having a baby," he continued. "Look at the surgery like the birth. Most people are mostly concerned about the actual process of the birth, when what they should be worried about is the next thirty or forty years of looking after the child." He grinned.

I had heard anecdotally that states like Colorado where there is a "no required helmet" ruling for motorcyclists resulted in more organs donors than other states. "Is that true?" I asked inquisitively.

"No, I have not heard that."

It's Not a Cure

As well as answering questions, he gave me more information than I could have ever wished for in terms of how lungs work, what the operation involves and how all they could offer was to exchange of one disease state for another. "It's not a cure," he emphasized several times.

"You would be exchanging one set of problems for another. I just want to make sure you understand that. And there are other potential complications. You will be more susceptible to certain forms of cancer, there may be damage to your kidneys, and there is the constant threat of rejection."

"But would I get my life back?" I asked nervously. He looked at me for a few moments as if contemplating the answer.

"Yes," he conceded at last. "It would give you your life back."

After a good ninety minutes with him, I felt like I had been given a grilling by a police interrogator on one of those crime shows on television. The only thing was that I wasn't sure if I had been talking to the good cop or the bad cop. And besides, the operation itself is not the part the doctors are most concerned about. No matter how horribly complex the mechanics seem to me (someone who shudders at the idea of changing the oil in his car), that's not the tricky part, apparently. The tricky part is the bit at the back end, where it's the whole rigmarole around the risk of rejection of the new organs that makes the doctors antsy.

If you think about it, our body is designed to repel foreign invaders. Our immune system does this spectacular job of roughing up any bugs that try to set up home in our bodies to stop us getting overwhelmed and sick. In most cases, our immune system forms this shield that keeps us safe from everyday bacteria and viruses that are all around. Remember "War of the Worlds" and how those aren't-we-so-darn-clever martians just plain forgot to defend themselves against the Earthly bacteria? And our immune system works for us twenty-four hours a day, seven days a week.

Problems start when we get run down, tired or stressed and our immune system gets compromised. The guards weaken and the bugs find a breach in the defenses to let in the invaders that make us ill. If it's a common cold, the immune system bounces back in a matter of days. If it's something more serious, a dose of common kitchen mould, also known as penicillin or antibiotics, gives us some extra help to kill the little devils. However, the best idea is usually to keep the immune system fit and strong to avoid a breach in the first place.

So how does that theory work when you introduce a whole new organ into the body? How do you stop the immune system from kicking its tiny sentries out of their bunks, mounting their bayonets on their muskets and yelling "Chaaarge!" when the last thing you want is for them to win?

The answer is a cocktail of chemicals that will attempt to find just the right balance between two competing forces. One side of the equation is pushing down the aggressive parts of the immune system that want to kick out the new lungs (xenophobia at its finest, by any other name). The other side of the equation is encouraging it to divert its nervous energy against the hooligan neighbor bugs that want to whack the body with mundane things like the common cold. That's where the natural immune system really gets put through a road test.

"So do you want to go ahead?" Lyu asked.

"Yes." Julie and I both answered and nodded our heads at the same time. We wanted to go ahead.

We felt like we didn't have a choice. I knew that by the very fact I was being interviewed by a lung transplant physician, and that lung transplant was a therapy of last resort, I had no choice but to move forward if I wanted to live.

What Did I Do to Deserve This?

Anyone who has been diagnosed with a serious illness goes through various stages of emotions. I was no exception. First, there was the stage of pure disbelief.

"I don't believe this can be happening. It all seems like a nightmare," I remember saying. "That isn't me; they must have made an error. Any minute now I am going to get a call from the hospital telling me it is all one big mistake. Any minute now I am going to wake up from this bad dream." But you don't wake up. It isn't a bad dream, just a really tough reality that you have to be strong enough to deal with.

Then there is the stage of denial. "I am not as ill as they say. Look, I can still walk, run and swim. I'm not ill. I can't be. It's probably just a bad cold. It will clear up any day now" So you just try and ignore the symptoms and hope that they will go away on their own. No such luck. The symptoms don't go away.

Then there is stage of introspection: the "why me?" question. "What did I do to deserve this"? I remember saying over and over. "I've never smoked and have always looked after my lungs. It is all so unfair." I could recall my grandmother, who smoked cigarettes all her life, living well into her eighties. If smoking was so bad for you, why did she always appear to be so fit and healthy? It was not that I begrudged her a life of health, but at the same time, I could not help feeling envious of her good fortune. It all seemed so unfair.

Then, gradually, there was the stage of acceptance. It took a long time before I accepted that I needed a lung transplant, and that there was really no alternative if I wanted to live. It took me even longer – several months, in fact – before I was emotionally ready to feel deeply grateful at being given a second chance at life.

I can't be too introspective in my feelings about being ill with the lung disease, as I wasn't the only one that it affected. My wife Julie bore the brunt of my condition, as she had to continue to live a normal family life, looking after our two children, while becoming increasingly concerned about me.

The diagnosis I received in 2004 really upset her. At the time, my outlook was bleak, as the most specialized pulmonologists we could find could only shrug their collective shoulders and hope that the condition would not get any worse. Julie could see my physical deterioration, and was aware of my cough and shortness of breath as a constant reminder that I was not getting better.

It is strange for a young woman to contemplate the death of her husband. "It's a conversation no one wants to have," she said. "Quite apart from the emotional trauma, there is the practical side: who is going to pay the bills and take out the trash."

Julie decided to support me for as long as it took and to never accept "no" for an answer. "We pushed on, regardless of the obstacles," she said. "We had done it before, when our son, Alex, was born, and we decided that we could do it again." Alex had been born ten weeks prematurely and needed a respirator for the first two weeks of his life.

Back at home, Julie and I talked together about what we had learned. There was such a barrage of information it was like being thrown into a new and unknown subject at university. Maybe in a few weeks that part will be clearer, we thought. We became very task-focused, just concentrating on the next test, or the next procedure, or the next pharmacy visit, and not looking much further into the future.

In the meantime, I was thinking, "It's just the lungs, just two lungs." Nice one. Thanks, Elaine.

CHAPTER 6

Work Up or Work Out?

After the consultation with Lyu, I was anxious to get on with the process of the work up that would determine my suitability as a candidate for a lung transplant. No one seemed to be questioning any longer if I should have a lung transplant; it seemed to just be a question of when.

The lung transplant coordinator at the University of Colorado Hospital was a calm, cheerful nurse called Maren. Her role was to coordinate the next steps by scheduling the battery of medical tests. The lung transplant coordinator is really a patient's lifeline in the process working up to the lung transplant, and well beyond. She is the first point of contact for prospective recipients, and coordinates all aspects, such as assimilating your records, your requests, your appointments, the feedback on outcomes and next steps. The lung transplant coordinator makes everything happen, and in many instances, your life literally hangs in her hands. She visits patients in the hospital just to check up on your progress after the operation and to advise you on what you can and cannot do (no alcohol or grapefruit juice, as they impede the absorption of the all-important medications).

She is the human face of what could be quite an impersonal process. As a patient, you are not just going through a series of steps, but you are going through a series of steps that are critical to your survival. The lung transplant coordinator recognizes the emotional rollercoaster that transplant patients are on, and is prepared for the tears, the elation and everything in between on that journey.

The work up of tests had a dual purpose. It was designed to ascertain if a patient was healthy enough, yet ill enough, to warrant going down the lung transplant route. It was a strange position to be in, almost hoping to be sick enough to be given the chance of a new life with new lungs, and hoping not to be so sick as to be disqualified from the procedure. In addition, the tests were designed to provide a road map for the surgeons to refer to when they were actually performing the transplant surgery.

The tests were scheduled for the week after the Thanksgiving holiday of 2007, and they were numerous and varied. There were fifteen or so:

Lung Transplant Work Up Tests

Pulmonary Function Test	Measures how well the lungs are working and determines the blood's capacity to carry oxygen. Patients will be asked to breath into various machines to determine results.
Ventilation and Perfusion Scan (VQ Scan)	Determines lung function. To measure ventilation (air flow), patients breathe into a mask while pictures are taken of the lungs. To measure perfusion (blood flow), dye is injected into the veins and pictures are taken.
Chest X-Ray	Provides a full picture of the heart and lungs. This helps to determine the amount of lung damage the lung disease has caused.
Echocardiogram (Echo)	Shows the function of the heart muscle and heart valves. Gel is placed on the patient's chest and an ultrasound machine is used to look at the heart.
Electrocardiogram (EKG or ECG)	Shows the pattern of electrical waves in the heart. A cardiologist interprets these patterns to evaluate how well the heart is working.
Multiple Gated Blood Pool Scan (MUGA)	Measures how well the left and right ventricles of the heart pump blood. A radioactive dye is injected into the veins and a machine takes pictures of the heart.

Cardiac Catheterization	Measures various pressures in the heart and lungs. Depending on age and medical history, dye may be injected into the arteries to study the coronary (heart) arteries. A catheter is placed in a large vessel in the groin or neck and advanced to your heart.
Blood Tests	Checks the blood count, blood and tissue type, blood chemistries, immune system function, and checks for certain infectious diseases
Tissue Typing	Determines blood type and genetic make up. These tests determine the compatibility between donor and recipient.
Noninvasive Vascular Studies	An ultrasound-like machine measures the blood flow in the carotid arteries (vessels that supply blood to the brain) and in the vessels in the legs.
Kidney Function Studies	Determine if the kidneys are working correctly. This involves blood tests and a twelve-hour urine collection.
Abdominal Ultrasound	Performed on patients forty years and older, or patients with a history of gallbladder disease, to check for gallstones or inflammation of the gallbladder.
CAT Scan (CT)	A scan that takes pictures of the lungs. These pictures help to determine which lung to transplant. The patient may also need a scan of the abdomen and pelvis.

Barium Enema (BE)	Performed on patients forty years and older to examine the large intestine and colon for disease, obstruction or bleeding. A type of dye is put through a rectal tube, and then X-ray and a scope are used to examine the large intestine and colon.
Colonoscopy	Performed on patients forty years and older to examine the lining of the rectum and colon. A tube is inserted into the rectum and lower colon and a scope is used to check for cancer.

The appointment with the hospital's financial officer was a high priority. Their role was simple: to review the patient's medical insurance policy, the terms and conditions and the fine print to ensure that the hospital would be paid. I was not anxious about going to this appointment, as I had medical insurance that specifically covered lung transplant, but at the same time, it is always a little nerve-wracking until you find out that you have cleared that most important hurdle.

My appointment didn't take long. I proffered the folder full of insurance documents to the grim faced official. After several minutes of silence as she flipped through the documents, she said "You're fine, you're well covered." I breathed a quiet sigh of relief. At least I didn't have to worry about the financial aspect of the ordeal.

"Out of interest," I said. "If I didn't have insurance, how much would a transplant cost?"

"But you do have insurance," she said, eyeing me suspiciously.

"Yes, I know. And I'm thankful for that. But say I didn't? How much would it cost to get a lung transplant?"

She looked at me coolly. "Before we would do a lung transplant, without insurance, we would require cleared funds, cash, of $250,000," she said, unemotionally. I wondered how often she had responded to that question to uninsured (or under-insured) potential patients who had no hope of coming up with such a sum.

As part of the work up assessment, I had to complete a six-minute-walk to help the physicians assess my lung capacity. For a marathon runner, it initially seemed laughable to me that I was going to be measured over the trivial distance that could be covered in six minutes. Walking at a brisk pace of four miles per hour, I should be able to walk around 0.4 of a mile in six minutes. When I reported to the nurse who was going to measure my progress, I half thought I would be taken outside to walk at a sprint pace around the parking lot.

But no. She indicated that I was to be measured walking up and down one of the short corridors, while towing my oxygen tank. It was one of these humbling moments when I had the sudden realization that I was not nearly as able as I had thought. I managed the first couple of laps without too much difficulty, but soon began to slow down, as my coughing started, and I felt more and more out of breath.

"This is ridiculous," I thought to myself. "I can go much faster than this."

"How much longer?" I asked the nurse through panting breath, thinking that the six minutes must have been up quite a few minutes ago.

"Just over three minutes left," she said, looking at her watch. "Just go as far as you can."

I was still determined to break the hospital speed record for the six-minute-walk, so I pushed on, and after what seemed like an hour of walking - but it was only six minutes - I finished the test, panting and coughing. I felt like I had just had a severe work out, and I gratefully sucked in the air through my cannula.

"That will do for now," said the nurse kindly, and she led me back to the waiting room.

We touched base regularly with Maren as the week of testing progressed. My brother John had come over from Scotland to help me out during this difficult period, and he did a splendid job driving me to the hospital each morning and escorting me from appointment to appointment. The tests were unpleasant, but I knew that they were necessary steps on the route that I was going down. I did not feel particularly well that week, as in addition to the testing, I had to pull around my oxygen tank to which I was tethered to give me the oxygen I needed to breathe.

There was a constant concern – on my part – that the oxygen might run out, and I was always glancing surreptitiously at the tank's gauge to determine how long it would be before I needed to change the tank. Indeed, John even went to the extent of buying a portable electricity generator that we kept in the garage in case there was a power outage at home and my oxygen concentrator stopped working.

Spare oxygen tanks were rolling around in the back of the car wherever we went, and we had to carry extras when we made the trip to the hospital. That made the whole routine more stressful than it would have been otherwise.

I spoke to Maren one day about some of the tests, and she made the comment that my CT scan "looked really good."

"What do you mean "really good," I asked cautiously, hardly daring to believe that the scan had revealed a healthy picture of my lungs. I had a silent hope that this whole process was one big mistake and that any day now one of the doctors would call me up and tell me that my lungs were just fine after all. But no, that wasn't happening.

"Well, by "really good", said Maren, a little embarrassed, "I mean that it looks good for getting you on the transplant list. Your lungs are in really bad shape."

"Any broccoli in there?" I asked.

"What do you mean?" Maren sounded confused.

"Well, I read somewhere that there was a man who had suffered respiratory problems for years, and doctors eventually found a sprig of broccoli stuck in one of his lungs."

"Eh, no, there's no broccoli," she said. That was my last grasp at the straw of an easy answer to my breathing difficulties.

By the end of the week, I was exhausted, but felt relieved that it was over. I felt that it was only a matter of a few days before I was put on the list for my transplant. Maren had told us that the average waiting time on the list was twelve to eighteen months. I don't know why, but I felt certain that I would be transplanted much sooner. All I needed to do was to get onto the list.

Do Over

As a first-timer to the process, and looking back, I underestimated the extent to which the thorough battery of tests I was being subjected to could result in my being disqualified as a patient. I believed that as I felt healthy and well – apart, of course, from my lungs – I would automatically be one of the strongest candidates for a transplant. It never crossed my mind that my medical condition would render me ineligible, in the view of the Lung Transplant Committee at the University of Colorado Hospital, for a lung transplant.

"Gavin, we need to run some of the tests again. Can you come in this week?" It was Maren on the phone, calling to tell me that I needed to come back in to the hospital.

A week had passed since the conclusion of the first wave of testing of the work up and Julie and I were waiting anxiously at home for word from the hospital. To be recalled for more testing was not what we were expecting.

"Everything's alright though, isn't it?" I heard Julie asking, when I passed the phone to her to speak to Maren. Yes, she assured us, we just need to rerun some of the tests to get a more accurate picture of a few critical areas.

So the next week – it was now the second week in December – I reluctantly reported back at the hospital for the additional tests. I was not particularly concerned by the recall. I just wanted the testing part to be over so that I could get on with the rest of the waiting.

Two weeks had passed since the rerun of the tests. We had not heard from Maren, but understood that my case was going to be put before the Transplant Committee any day. We were anxious to know the result, and how quickly I would be put on the list.

We were at home again. The phone rang. "Mr. Maitland? It's Dr. Lyu from the University of Colorado Hospital. Do you have a minute?" As soon as I answered the phone, I knew by the tone of his voice and the fact that he was calling me "Mr. Maitland" as opposed to "Gavin" that all was not well. It was Friday, December 21st, 2007, four days before Christmas.

"Mr. Maitland," Dr. Lyu went on, "We have a problem. I think it is unlikely that we are able to do your transplant."

"What do you mean?" I gulped, scarcely able to comprehend what he had just said.

"Well, there is a complicated pattern of collateral blood vessels around your lungs that have formed to compensate for the scale of your disease. It means your chest wall has many blood vessels that are not normally there. Our surgeons are concerned that there is a high risk that you will bleed to death on the operating table if we perform the surgery." He paused.

"Is there nothing you can do?" I stammered. I couldn't think of what to say. I couldn't believe what I was hearing.

"Well, we could go back and look at your case again, I suppose." Lyu sounded reluctant. "I could discuss it again with the surgeons."

"Could you do that…please?" I could feel my voice fading off, as my stomach filled with dread.

"Okay, I will call you back on Wednesday," he said and rung off. He sounded like it was another day in the office for him.

Essentially, we had to wait until Wednesday, December 26th - the day after Christmas – to hear back from Dr. Lyu. Not surprisingly, we had a miserable Christmas. Julie's parents, Larry and Henna, as well as my mum, May, were staying with us, helping look after Alex and Riley. When I told them about the telephone conversation with Lyu, there were a lot of tears. It seemed particularly harsh that we were left dangling right through the holiday period until the following Wednesday. We waited with great trepidation as the days crawled by.

Alex and Riley were great – as always. In fact, their positive attitude throughout the whole lung transplant adventure was an important source of inspiration and strength. We had decided early on in the process to be as honest with them as possible and to tell them what was going on, but not to scare them. They were very nonchalant about the fact that their Dad spent most of the day lying on the couch or in bed.

Riley, my beautiful six-year-old daughter, used to say "Hey, Dad, I can always find you in the house without calling for you, I just follow the tubes!" To her, the tubes served a useful purpose beyond providing oxygen. She often matter-of-factly mentioned to her friends at school that her "Daddy was waiting for a lung transplant," as if it was the most normal thing in the world. Alex, aged eight, was quieter about the whole thing. He would not ask any questions, but he still enjoyed spending time with me, and would often lie up against me and read his book when I was lying down. I tried to reassure him that everything was going to be alright, and he would just look at me. I think he understood much more than we gave him credit for.

When Wednesday eventually rolled around, I couldn't wait for Lyu to call. I called him at 8:30 a.m., got his voice mail, and left a message to call me back. He called back at 4:30 p.m. I saw on the caller ID that it was the University of Colorado Hospital on the line, so I pusillanimously passed the phone over to Julie to answer.

Julie took the phone and spoke to Lyu. She didn't say much during the five minute call. She nodded a lot, and I could tell by her expression that there had not been any breakthrough. Eventually, her expression turned weary, and she hung up.

"What did he say?"

"He gave me all sorts of reasons why they don't want to do the transplant on you," she said. "Apparently, they are now also concerned that your right diaphragm is paralyzed, and so won't be any good to your new lungs anyway." She looked at me and started to cry. There was more.

"He also said…" she sobbed, "that if this was his family, he would start looking for another transplant center."

So that was the end of our contact with the University of Colorado Hospital. We never did receive any kind of official notification that we were not being considered by them any more, nor any specific reason that they would not perform the surgery. They just stopped communicating with us. The only reason I can speculate about for their refusal was that they lacked the surgical expertise to take on a particularly challenging case. However, if this was the case, I would have preferred a straight answer from them rather than just being cut adrift.

I still entertained hopes that they would somehow change their minds, although Julie knew right away that we had to look for an alternative – and fast.

If You Can Keep Your Head…

The poet Rudyard Kipling once wrote "If you can keep your head when all about you are losing theirs and blaming it on you…"

That is what Julie did. She lost no time, keeping a cool head while almost everyone else, myself included, descended into despair and panic. It sounds ridiculous now, but I had not considered the possibility that I would be turned down by the hospital for transplant surgery, and I had not thought of any contingency plan if I needed to go elsewhere.

On the contrary, Julie's first thought was: "where else can we go?" And she started the quest right away. She got on the internet and started looking at transplant centers all across the United States. She even considered centers in Canada and the United Kingdom. We were well aware we were working to a deadline, as my lung disease was obviously progressing. Three months before, I could walk, albeit slowly, without oxygen. Now I could barely lie still on my bed without my oxygen supply.

By the weekend, with the help of several personal contacts with pulmonary physicians and other specialists, Julie had compiled a list of the top twenty-two transplant centers in the United States, which we evaluated for the most experience in the transplant of lungs with complex fibrotic conditions.

Looking back, we probably should have targeted the top five centers first, but we knew that time was a precious commodity and that each center may take days or weeks to evaluate and respond to the information. We collected my medical records from the University of Colorado Hospital records department and made twenty-two copies of all the paperwork and compact disks with the various scans. Julie had made several telephone and email requests to Dr. Lyu to write a covering letter to summarize his findings. Once we eventually got it, Julie described it as "the world's most depressing letter" as it spelled out the medical condition and practically said that there was no hope of a lung transplant or recovery. We had no choice but to shrug it off and focus on the task at hand. By the end of the weekend, we had sent the twenty-two packages by FedEx Priority Overnight to the various centers.

From her work as a medical communications specialist, Julie was also on first name terms with several leading pulmonologists in different parts of the United States. She did not hesitate to call them up and ask for their opinions: "If it was your family member, where would you send them for a lung transplant?" she would ask.

Three transplant programs came to the fore: the University of Pittsburgh Medical Center, the Cleveland Clinic and Duke University Medical Center. We discovered quickly that the University of Pittsburgh would not accept my brand of medical insurance (but helpfully offered to go ahead with an upfront deposit of $500,000 in cash), so the list was quickly shortened further to the Cleveland Clinic or Duke University Medical Center.

The reputation of Duke clinched the deal for me, as well as the average waiting time for organs. We had contact with other institutions that had called or written to us following receipt of the FedEx package with my medical records. In our 'interviews' with some of the centers by telephone, I clearly recall several of the centers telling me how good their transplant programs were because "our surgeons were trained at Duke."

After you hear that for the third or fourth time, you start thinking: why don't I just go to Duke? Cindy Lawrence, the lung transplant coordinator we had been talking to from Duke said that the average waiting time on the list at Duke was a mere twenty-one days. This short time seemed incredible, especially when I had been quoted an average waiting time of twelve to eighteen months by the University of Colorado. I just needed to get on the list.

Waiting Times

I still don't understand how the quoted average waiting times can vary so drastically between transplant institutions. How was it that that the team at the University of Colorado Hospital believed that I would wait for up to a year for new lungs, while the team at Duke University could predict that the average time on the waiting list would be twenty-one days?

Part of the answer probably lies in the geographical partitioning of the United States for the purposes of allocating organs to people on the waiting list. There are eleven geographical regions in the United States, and I can only believe that in the region where Duke University Medical Center is located, the number of organ donors as a percentage of the general population is quite favorable, as opposed to the region in which the University of Colorado Hospital is located. The data provided by UNOS, the United Network for Organ Sharing, a federally mandated organization, shows that there were 169 lung transplants in the Duke University region in 2008 and 318 available organs, which means that that region is in the immensely fortunate position of having more organs available than are in demand.

The other factor might be the policy that individual institutions follow when placing potential organ recipients onto the waiting list. It seemed to me that the University of Colorado Hospital, after reviewing the results of a work up, would place a potential recipient onto the waiting list, regardless of the proximity of the procedures (i.e. regardless of how far or close to death they were). By contrast, it seems that Duke University had a policy of only placing a potential recipient onto the list when they were in the critical zone (i.e. sick enough to warrant getting a lung transplant, but well enough to survive the procedure). These differences may account for the differences in quoted and actual waiting times on the list.

There was a direct flight from Denver to Raleigh-Durham, and I saw on the internet that the temperature in North Carolina at that time of year was in the seventies. I made up my mind. Two weeks into January, I said to Julie, "Let's go to Duke."

As they already had my medical records, Julie called them back and arranged for an appointment for my work up. I was a little downhearted to hear from the lung transplant coordinator, Cindy Lawrence, that Duke was going to make me go through the entire battery of tests again despite having my records from the University of Colorado Hospital. Although, time would show that Duke were entirely right in electing to go through all the testing again, at that moment, I felt like they were unnecessarily repeating work that had already been done.

We got the appointment for the second week in February of 2008. I had to get through the next two weeks at home, while I waited for the appointment to come around.

Inspirations

Someone once advised me to read as many autobiographies and biographies as possible about inspiring people who had overcome seemingly impossible circumstances. The purpose was not to look *up to* the individuals, but to look *into* them and to explore their sources of strength. That is what I did during that four month period between starting to use supplemental oxygen and going to Duke. I wanted to get all the inspiration and mental toughness possible.

Among the books I read were Nelson Mandela's autobiography, a biography about Franklin D. Roosevelt, Lance Armstrong's "It's Not About The Bike," and Victor Frankel's traumatic "Man's Search for Meaning." All the books provided me with great encouragement and guidance on how to overcome physical hardship or life-threatening medical conditions. Nelson Mandela had the resolve and mental toughness to go through more than twenty-seven years of his life imprisoned by the South African authorities for his beliefs about the rights of his fellow South Africans. In his fascinating autobiography, "Long Walk To Freedom", I was continually amazed by his mental fortitude, his determination, and his never-varying belief that he was right and would be proved right in the end. I took a lot of inspiration from his example, and thought about him often when I was feeling down or depressed.

Even before imprisonment, Nelson Mandela faced many challenges. He recounted how he watched his father die from lung disease when he was a nine-year-old boy.

"I found him in my mother's hut, lying on the floor, in the midst of what seemed like an endless fit of coughing. Even to my young eyes, it was clear that my father was not long for this world. He was ill with some type of lung disease, but it

was not diagnosed, as my father had never visited a doctor. He remained in the hut for several days without moving or speaking, and then one night he took a turn for the worse."

He asked for his tobacco pipe, but his wife would not give it to him.

"But he persisted in calling for it, and eventually Nodayimani [his wife] *filled his pipe, lit it, and then handed it to him. My father smoked and became calm. He continued smoking for perhaps an hour, and then, his pipe still lit, he died."*

Franklin D. Roosevelt suffered from a total and permanent paralysis from the waist down from the age of thirty-nine until he died at the age of sixty-three. It was thought at the time that he suffered from polio. But he refused to believe that he was a permanent paraplegic and skillfully concealed his disability so that millions of Americans never knew he was confined to a wheelchair.

After his diagnosis, he went on to become governor of New York and to be elected an unprecedented four times as president. He remains the only US president to have served more than two terms. He courageously used the power of office and his personality to champion the fight against polio and make it a national cause. I found it particularly inspiring that he refused to give up in the face of his incurable disease and fought on to achieve his dreams.

Lance Armstrong, the professional cyclist, provided me with a modern day inspirational athletic story. He not only survived testicular cancer, where a tumor metastasized to his brain and lungs, but he went on to win the Tour de France cycling race an unprecedented seven times. The prognosis from his surgery was originally very depressing, and he underwent cancer treatments for brain and testicular surgery, including chemotherapy. I found his story to be inspirational due to his indomitable spirit and his willingness to fight to get back to his athletic best. It is important to mention that he had his down days as well when he was in the midst of his treatment, or when he found it difficult to get back on his bike, but his strength of spirit pulled him through the dark periods.

Victor Frankel's book, "Man's Search for Meaning," gave me an enormous boost in helping me keep my perspective on what was happening to me. Frankel, an Austrian Jewish neurologist and psychiatrist, was a prisoner of the Nazis for two and a half years during World War Two. His book chronicles his experiences as an inmate in the concentration camp, as well as his analysis about the prisoners' attempts to find meaning among their atrocious living conditions.

I remember reading a passage where the prisoners were forced to stand to attention outside their miserable huts in the middle of the night in minus twenty degree Fahrenheit conditions. And all without shoes. The inhumanity of their treatment is barely credible. I remember being in Denver in the early winter days of 2008, when the temperature outside was minus twenty degrees Fahrenheit. The only difference was that I was in a warm house at the time. Examples like that really helped put everything into perspective for me as I moved closer to the lung transplant.

Victor Frankel quotes the phrase from the German philosopher, Nietzsche that he used in the concentration camp: *"Was mich nicht umbringt, macht mich stärker"* (that which does not destroy/kill me, makes me stronger). I decided then and there to adopt this attitude, and indeed I now include the saying in all of my email correspondence.

CHAPTER 7

Heading To North Carolina

It was difficult to leave home for the four-hour flight to Raleigh-Durham in North Carolina. Julie was coming with me, but we were leaving Alex and Riley at home, in the capable hands of Julie's mom, Henna, and my mum, May. We decided that it was really important to us to ensure that the kids kept up at school and their various activities and that there was as much continuity as possible in their lives. Leaving the children was tough, as Julie and I had never been apart from them for more than a few days at one time. We had a tearful goodbye, and I told them I would be back soon with sparkling new lungs.

My elder brother, William, had come over from London to visit us for a couple of days, and his visit coincided with a visit from my long-time friend, Marc Bozon, who had travelled all the way from the Netherlands. I have known Marc for over fifteen years, and he has three children around the ages of Alex and Riley. We got to spend less than forty-eight hours together before Julie and I had to leave, but it raised my spirits a lot to have him and my brother there.

The flight was complicated due to the fact that I had to travel with supplementary oxygen. We had to arrange to leave the portable oxygen tanks at the airport on my departure, use the on-board oxygen on the United Airlines flight while flying, then pick up the pre-arranged portable oxygen bottles on arrival at Raleigh-Durham.

The flight attendant on the flight was very helpful during the four hour journey. He asked what was wrong that I needed the supplementary oxygen. When I told him that I was going for a lung transplant, he said, "I didn't know that they could do that." My grim, unspoken response to that was "A few short months before, I didn't know that they could do that either." I just hoped that the specialists at Duke could help me where the University of Colorado Hospital had not.

We arrived in North Carolina without incident and caught a taxi, along with four tanks of oxygen, to the Marriott Residence Inn, which would be our home for the next few months. The hotel is a twenty minute drive away from Duke University Medical Center, a good thing, because my evaluation appointments began at 8:00 a.m. on Monday morning.

Another difficult, slow week followed. We made sure we were on time for every appointment and every interview. We met my designated transplant pulmonologist, Dr. Steele, a serious, thoughtful man, and my lung transplant coordinator, Cindy Lawrence. The staff at Duke was phenomenally helpful in getting me from appointment to appointment, while Julie and I dealt with moving around with supplementary oxygen. At this point, I could barely walk, even with the assistance of the oxygen, so Julie had to push me around in a hospital wheel chair.

It soon became clear why Duke University was redoing many of the tests that had already been performed by the University of Colorado Hospital. Duke's physicians only had confidence in testing that was done by their own team in their own location.

"We don't see a lot of the complications that were highlighted by the University of Colorado," Dr. Steele said. "I expect you will be transplanted within three weeks."

I was delighted that he seemed so confident I was a good candidate for transplant. It seemed that the surgeons at Duke University took a certain pride in accepting difficult or complicated surgical cases that other medical institutions may have turned down. However, even though I was pleased and relieved, it also made me a little nervous that we were moving so fast towards the transplant itself. I knew in my heart that it was essential for me to get the operation, but at the same time, I was understandably nervous at the thought of being cut open and having my lungs removed from my body and replaced with a new set.

Running Out of Time…

During one of the tests during the week, Julie had a side conversation with one of the pulmonologists. She broached the topic of how much time was left. This was a topic I had always avoided, as I didn't want to hear someone's opinion – even an informed opinion of one of the pulmonologists – about how long it was before I died.

There always seemed to be an element of self-fulfilling prophecy in these types of predictions; in my opinion, if you are convinced that you are going to die, then your chances of surviving are minimal.

I recall reading on one of the hospital's websites that they would not consider lung transplant until the patient had less than two years to live. I also knew that lung transplant – like any organ transplant – was a medical therapy of last resort when the patient had run out of all other options. So I knew I was in the 'end of life' category, but I still didn't really believe it, in spite of everything I had been through. "He can probably go until June without a lung transplant, but not much longer," Julie was told. It was February so that meant four months. Julie didn't tell me that particular piece of information until quite a bit after my transplant, but she knew that we did not have a lot of time. Nevertheless, although I didn't know the exact time frame, I was acutely aware of how I felt. And I felt that my lung functionality was deteriorating at an alarming rate.

At the early stages of my lung disease, I didn't notice how much weight I was losing or my impaired lung function, as the deterioration was gradual and I was living with it every day. Now, in February of 2008, I could tell by the physical activities that I could not do that I was deteriorating more rapidly than before. Even the shortest of walks would send me into a spasm of coughing, which in turn, sent my oxygen saturation level down in to the eighty percentage zone. That in turn left me highly susceptible to a heart attack, due to the sudden increased workload put on my cardiovascular system.

Even though Julie would often say encouragingly that I was "going to be around for a long time yet," I did find myself contemplating my own death, which is a strange experience. My biggest fear was not for myself, but the fact that I would be leaving Julie and my two beautiful children, Alex and Riley. Being a father to Alex and Riley has been the most rewarding and worthwhile experience of my life. I treasure every moment with them, and revel in their funniness and wonder about the world. There were so many things that I wanted to experience with them that I could not bear to think about not being with them.

One of the many great things about children is their unfailing belief in everything turning out for the best. Alex and Riley never doubted for a second that I would get my new lungs and would be soon be back to full health. They even made lists of "things we will do with Daddy when he gets home." The list included playing outside on their bikes, playing soccer, and taking walks with the dog. Both of them would often start a sentence with "When Daddy gets his new lungs…" They never doubted for a moment that the outcome would be positive. That is quite a lesson in itself for positive thinking.

Julie and I had a tough time – not to mention Alex himself – when Alex was born. He arrived ten weeks prematurely, and had to be delivered through an emergency cesarean section. He was hospitalized for seven weeks after his traumatic birth until he was big enough to go home. There were many moments in the first days and weeks of his precious new life when Julie and I were not sure that he would survive. But he fought back – his birth sign was Taurus, the determined bull – and has grown into a perfectly normal, healthy young man. To this day, I feel like I have a special attachment to my son, and cannot bear it to see him upset or hurt. But boys will be boys and he gets his fair share of cuts, bruises and scrapes, which I have to deal with on my own emotional level.

Riley is her own special person, very independent and quick-witted. She finds that things come to her very easily; at school, in sports and with her friends. The idea of leaving Julie, Alex, and Riley made me cry with frustration every time I thought about it.

On The List!

By the following Tuesday, I got a phone call from Cindy Lawrence.

"You'll be on the list by tomorrow, latest Thursday," she informed me. We just need to fill out some UNOS paperwork and you're there. Congratulations!"

I felt like crying with relief as I hugged Julie. I had done it; at last I was on the list.

My surgeon was a youthful-looking man called Dr. Duane Davies. My first meeting with him was in the weeks running up to my transplant. He had the reputation of being a brilliant transplant surgeon, but rather curt at the same time.

Julie and I had an appointment to see him one afternoon at his office at the Duke Clinic just after I was accepted on to the list, the weighted score assessment that allowed the medical staff to decide who would get the next available organs.

As he strode into the small clinic room, I could see that he was not one for light-hearted humor. I was still on oxygen, so it was not always easy to speak with the cannula on my nose. There was something comical about the close proximity we all found ourselves in that cramped room. Dr. Davies nodded curtly to acknowledge us, then immediately started with "Right, I'm going to scare you."

And scare us he did. He started with a fifteen minute monologue about all the things that could go wrong with the lung transplant operation, including, but not limited to, the fact that the operation might take up to twelve hours, I might be in hospital for up to four months after the operation, and that I might bleed to death during the procedure.

As I had been made aware during the extensive work up conducted prior to me being placed on the list, my lungs had begun to develop in an unusual way due to my lung disease. My body had "grown" extra blood vessels in the chest cavity to allow my body to get as much oxygen as possible, which meant that the blood vessels had begun to attach themselves to my chest wall.

Consequently, the operation to remove the lungs would involve cutting away these blood vessels before the old lungs could be removed. The process of severing the blood vessels would involve additional risk for excessive bleeding.

He wound up the meeting by asking us how long we had been married. I replied that it was almost ten years. "Well, that's good," he said, dryly. "It will take all your resilience to get through this."

Julie and I left the meeting with Dr. Davies in a daze. From our research, we knew a lot of the risks that were associated with the lung transplant process, and that my transplant was going to be riskier than most due to the blood vessel complication. But I felt sure that the fact that I was only forty-one years old, and had been in excellent physical health prior to my lung disease must count a lot in my favor.

I also felt that Dr. Davies had been unnecessarily downbeat in his assessment. I understood that doctors cannot gloss over medical evidence and have to call it as they see it, but I found the "whole truth" experience to be quite upsetting. Julie and I went out to the car, where Julie's dad, Larry, was waiting for us. I couldn't help it. I felt a sudden rush of despair and burst into tears.

With hindsight, I should have been ecstatic that the discussion with Dr. Davies had focused on the problems of the surgery, as opposed to if it could be done at all. Dr. Davies knew that I had been turned down by the University of Colorado Hospital as a candidate for lung transplant. He was not too interested in why I had been turned down, only that I presented a challenging case for him. He seemed to relish the challenge. He commented that his team at Duke often got the difficult cases that other transplant centers would not, or could not, accept.

Dry Runs

One thing that I had not anticipated – yet another thing – was the concept of dry runs. A dry run is where you are called and told that a matching set of lungs is available, and that you need to report to hospital immediately, but for some reason, the lungs are deemed no good, and the transplant does not go ahead. I had three dry runs before the real thing.

The first call came within twenty-four hours of being put on the transplant list. When my cell phone rang it was just after midnight. I grabbed the phone, which was at my bedside.

"Gavin? It's Katrina from lung transplant. Good news. We have a match for you. Nothing to eat or drink. You can come in through the ER."

Julie and I jumped out of bed. I felt a rush of excitement and nervousness at the same time. This was it. It was really happening.

It took us less than five minutes to get dressed and dash out to the car. Julie drove quickly along the deserted highway and we got to the hospital in less than 20 minutes. On the way, we called our parents on our cell phones to alert them to what was happening.

We entered the hospital through the emergency room and, once the receptionist had established why I was there, we were shown up to a room on the step down pulmonology unit on the seventh floor.

The nurses kicked into a well-organized routine as soon as I arrived at the unit. Before long, I had showered with special anti-bacterial soap, changed into a hospital gown, and had an intravenous site set up in my arm. Doctors began coming in with consent forms, which I was asked to sign. They were very clear on all the things that could go wrong during the operation: all the complications that might arise, the risks of permanent disability and worse.

I felt like asking them to emphasize all the aspects that could go right with the surgery, but I realized that they were only doing their jobs. The anesthesiologist came in to see me and to reassure me that they would do everything they could to ensure a successful outcome.

Then we had to wait. No one could tell us how long we would wait. It depended on a number of factors. The first one was how far away the organs were coming from. Duke had its own helicopter that took off and landed on the helipad on the roof of the hospital. As the nurse informed us, when a person was declared to be brain-dead, and the family had given the consent to him or her being an organ donor, a match for the organs was established through the UNOS system.

Once a match had been established – based on the criteria of blood type and physical size of the organs – the hospitals are contacted to prepare for the transplants.

At that point, the organs had not been examined by surgeons to determine their viability for use as transplant organs. This could generally only be done once the organs are removed from the donor's body. Usually, the lungs are among the last organs to be removed from the donor's body after other solid organs such as the heart, kidneys and liver. Then once the surgeons make an initial assessment that the lungs are viable, they are recovered and transported in an iced cooler as quickly as possible to the recipient's hospital.

The recipient – me, in this case – had to wait until the lungs actually arrived at the hospital. The lungs had been inspected and passed by a surgeon who traveled with the helicopter to the donor hospital, and they were re-examined by the chief surgeon at the recipient hospital to ensure that they were in good enough condition for transplant. If and only if they were declared to be in good enough condition would the patient be transferred to the pre-op area.

We had waited for four hours in the pulmonology unit when the phone rang. It was the lung transplant coordinator, Katrina, who told us that the lungs were no good, and I could go home again.

It is difficult to describe the emotional let down that I felt when I heard that the lungs were no good. It was like the sudden deflation of a vast balloon that is ready for take-off. However, as Julie pointed out, I would rather wait and get a pair of lungs that was in 100 percent good shape rather than a pair that was damaged.

In the three weeks while I was on the list, I participated in the pre-operative program at the Center for Living. Participating in both pre-and post-operative rehabilitation is a central tenet of Duke's transplant philosophy, and patients are required to start "working out" at the center as soon as they come to Duke – no matter what condition they are in. In my case, "exercising" at the Center for Living, even in my impaired state, certainly helped me make it through the difficult and emotionally draining waiting period. Although I was on oxygen, I could make my way round the track under my own steam, albeit with a steel oxygen tank on wheels dragging behind me. If I ever ran low on oxygen, I only had to signal to one of the respiratory therapists, and they would come over and change my tank. In this way, I could exercise as much as possible to keep myself fit and ready for the trauma of the imminent transplant surgery.

Other patients who had already had their surgery were a good source of information for those of us who were waiting. For the first few days, the newly transplanted patients were a little spaced out due to the drugs they were on, but they gradually became more coherent. I asked all kinds of questions: how long were you in the ICU, how quickly did you walk, was it painful, what was the worst part? All the information helped me to prepare for what was to come.

One of transplant recipients was Jeff, who had received his lung transplant just weeks before me. When Jeff arrived back at the Center for Living, he was ashen-faced, but walked determinedly upright. There was a tendency for new transplant patients to stoop forward a little to compensate for their surgical wounds, but Jeff stood tall.

Jeff was an enormous source of encouragement. He looked better and better each day that passed following his transplant. As we got to know each other better, he shared his harrowing story with me (see Chapter 13), which again made me realize how fortunate I was.

More Dry Runs

There were two more dry run calls over the next two weeks. Both times, I reported to the hospital as quickly as I could and went through all the surgical preparation, only to be informed that the lungs were no good. The second dry run lasted for over twenty hours, while we waited in the hospital for the phone to ring. That was an experience that was exhausting both physically and mentally for all of us. My dad had flown over to North Carolina from Scotland for a quick four-day visit, and he accompanied us to the hospital and through the tense wait of the third dry run.

To relieve the stress of the situation, Julie and her dad made the exciting discovery that the hospital cafeteria served freshly made delicious omelets at 3:00 a.m. Of course, I couldn't eat anything, so I had to sit irritably on my bed, waiting for them to return from their feasting.

Then came the fourth call, twenty-two days after I was put on the list: my cell phone rang at 6:30 p.m. on Thursday evening as I was lying on my bed in the hotel room, breathing oxygen from the omnipresent tube.

"Gavin? It's Cindy from lung transplant. Good news. We have a match for you. Nothing to eat or drink. Just come to the main reception at the hospital."

I was sure that this was the time for me. It's funny how you get an intuitive feeling when something is going to happen but, after three dry runs, I was sure that it was going to happen this time.

Julie drove me to the hospital in record time – if we had been stopped by a traffic cop, I would have had a really good excuse – and we went to reception to check in.

I felt very elated and very nervous at the same time – elated because I believed that my chance was here to receive the gift of a new set of lungs that would save my life. But at the same time I was nervous about the intense and life-threatening surgery that I was going to go through. Butterflies churned through my stomach, but nothing was going to stop me now. I was determined to go ahead.

Two hours later, I was lying in a bed in the pulmonary unit, showered, blood checked and the intravenous needle in my arm, when the phone rang. It was 2:00 a.m.

The Lungs Are Good

"Gavin, everything is fine. The lungs are good, we are ready to go," said the voice. I sank back and let out a sigh of relief. This was it: we were ready to go. I kissed Julie as two nurses wheeled me out of the pulmonology ward and into the pre-op area.

After so much waiting, everything seemed to move very quickly. I recall the intense activity of the nurses and doctors all around me, as they prepared for the surgery. I remember noticing how warm the whole room felt as I lay there on the trolley. As I didn't have my glasses on, the nurses and doctors around me were out of focus. The intravenous needle in my arm was connected to a sedative, which flowed quickly into my veins.

I was surprised by the speed of the whole process. After all the waiting, I was glad it was moving quickly, but at the same time, I was anxious about feeling so out of control. What could I do but leave everything in the hands of the experts, and trust that everything was going to be fine? I focused on the fact that I was going to wake up in what would seem like mere minutes with a perfect set of lungs. I closed my eyes as the anesthetic did its work and I slipped into unconsciousness.

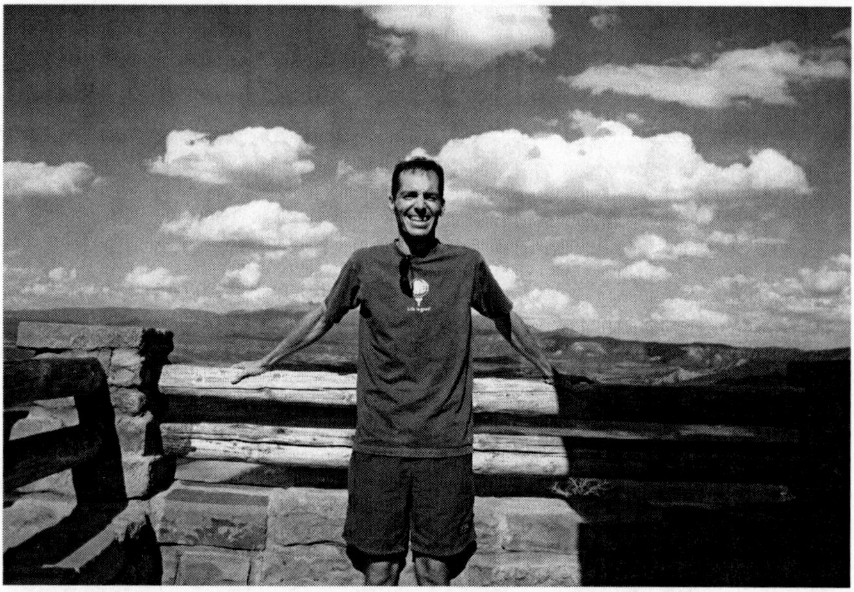

Near Durango in October 2007. I had lost so much weight that when my daughter, Riley, saw this picture recently she asked, "Who's that?"

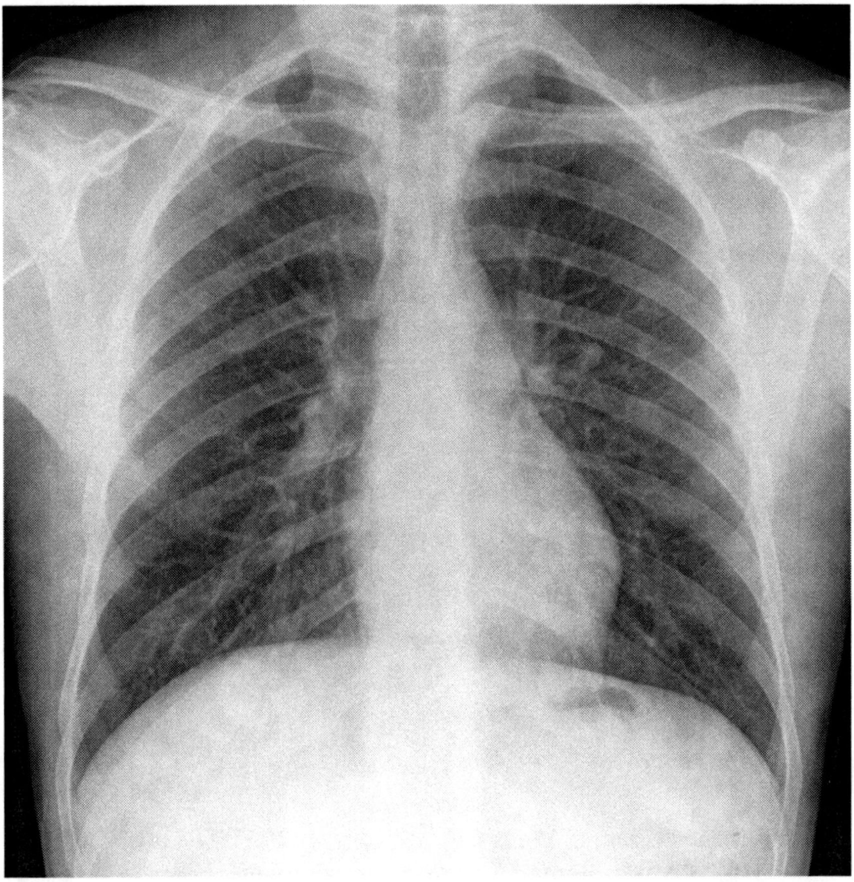

A chest x-ray of a normal adult healthy male. The heart in the center is of normal size and the lungs are clear.

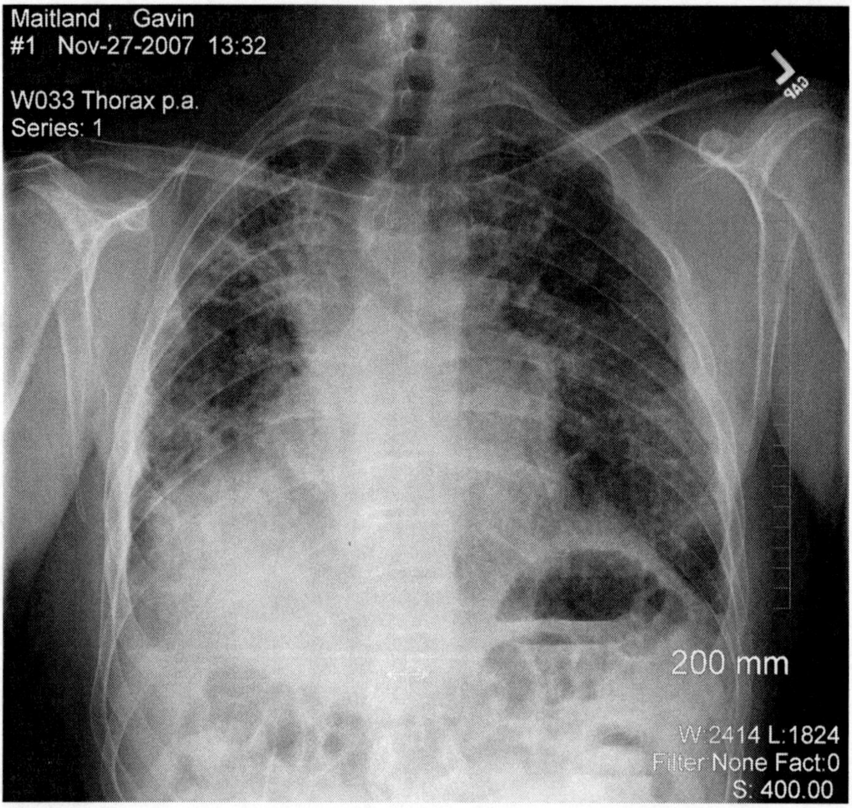

An x-ray of my diseased lungs from November 2007. The medical notes euphemistically commented "extensive abnormalities persist."

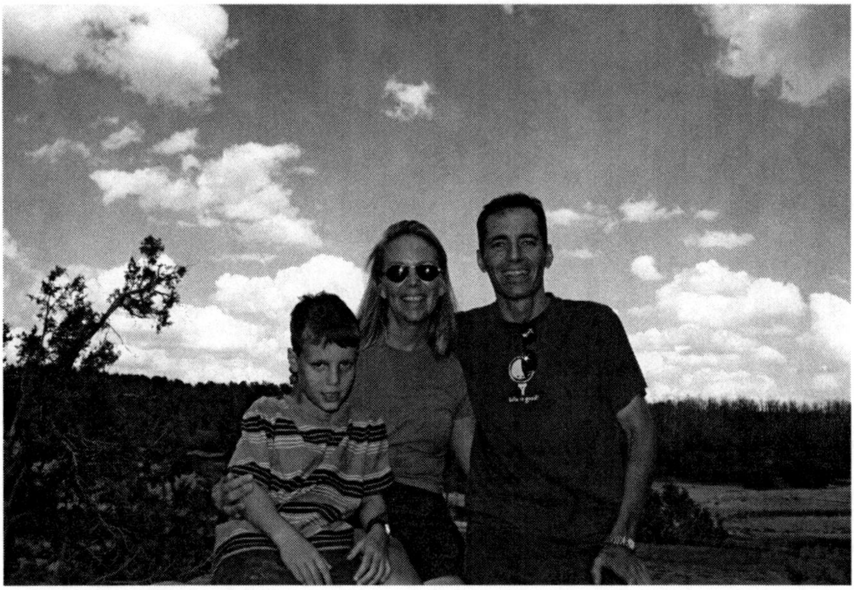

Alex, Julie and myself outside Durango. I weighed in at 125 lbs, compared to my usual 175 lbs.

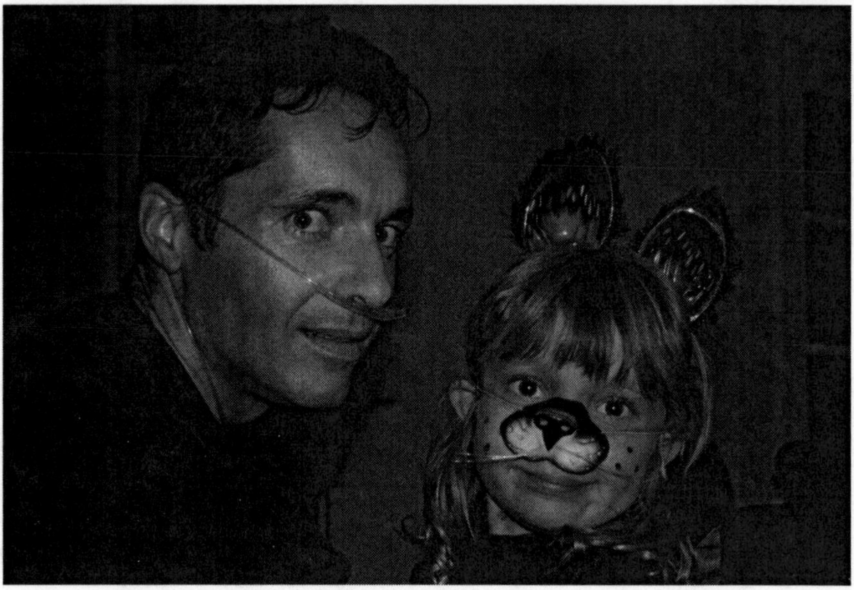

On oxygen, with Riley, at Halloween in October 2007.

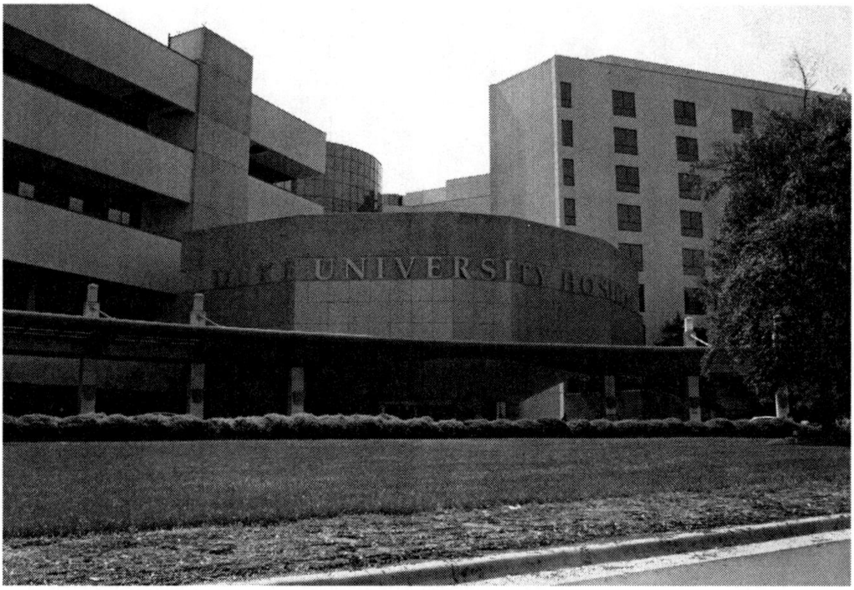

Duke University Hospital.

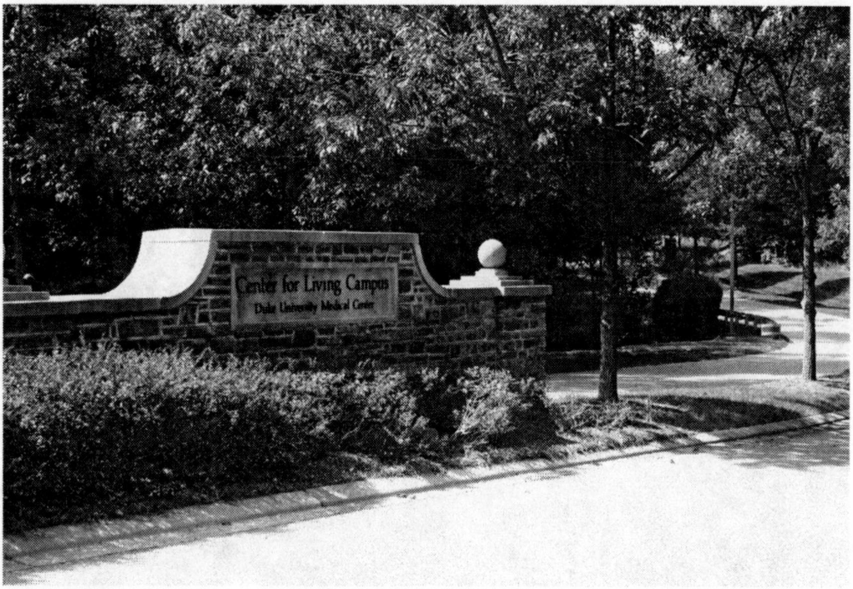

The Center for Living at Duke University Medical Center.

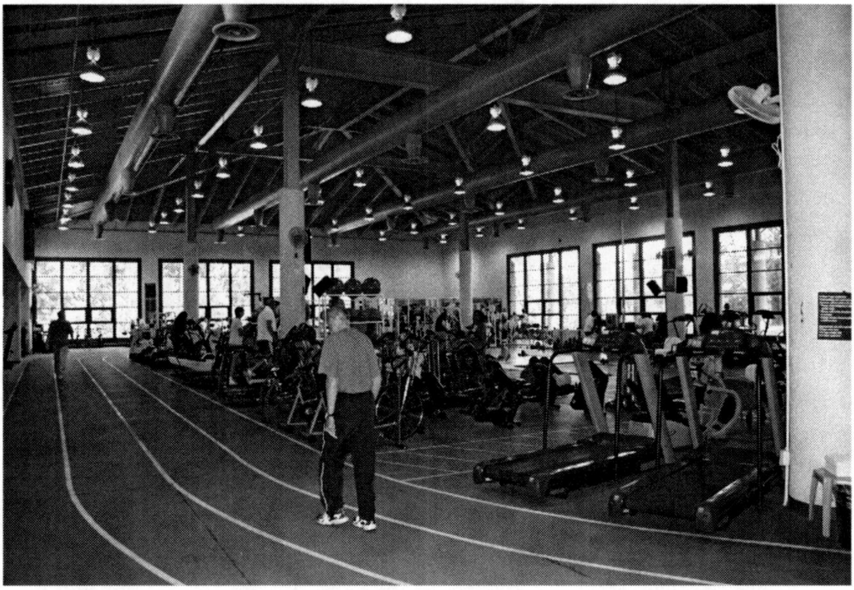

The track and exercise equipment at the Center for Living.

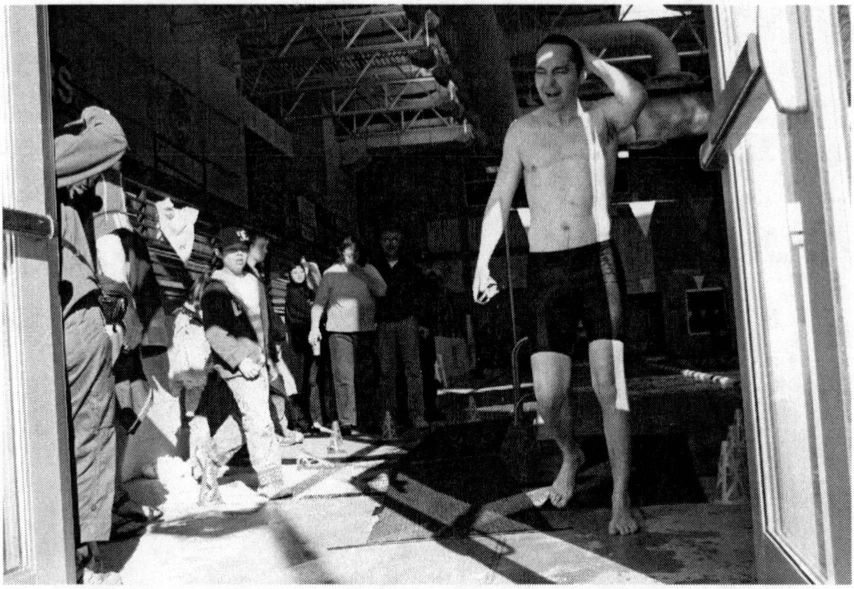

Leaving the pool at the end of the swimming leg of the Colorado School of Mines triathlon in April 2009.

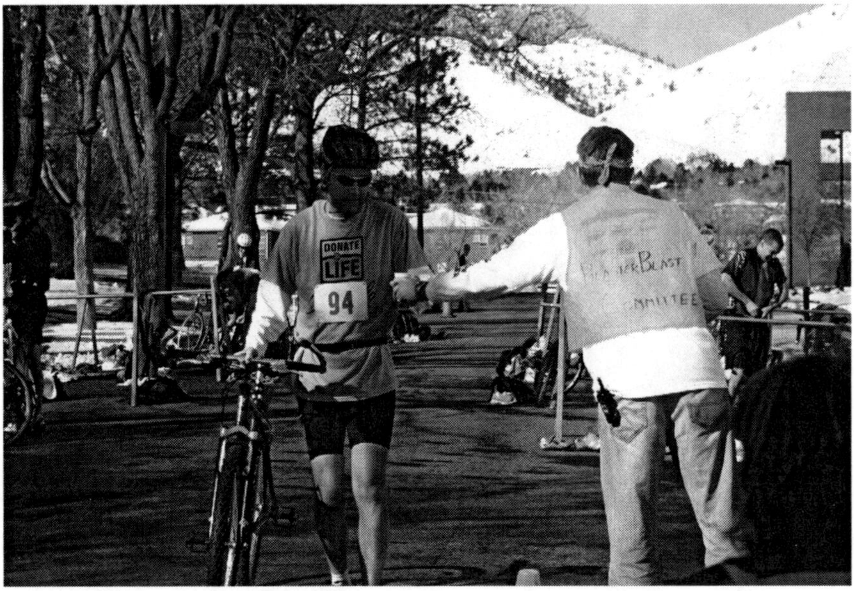

Starting the biking leg of the triathlon.

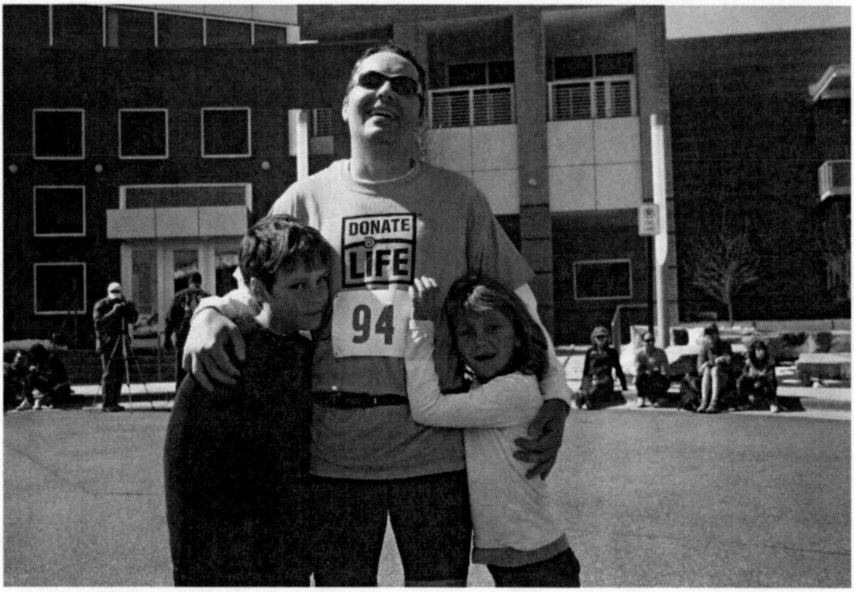

At the finish line of the triathlon with my biggest supporters, Alex and Riley.

CHAPTER 8

Recovery

Any stay in the hospital is unpleasant. You must give up privacy and accept that your body is there to be examined, poked or prodded at pretty much any time of the day or night. If you are positive, you will look at the experience as a period of healing and regeneration. If you're realistic, you will want to get out of there as soon as possible. For me, one of the worst things was being alone much of the time to think and imagine the worst case scenarios. It was during times like this that I first began to learn to "breathe and let go" – to accept the blessing of a new pair of lungs and to appreciate the simpler things in life – like the ability to be able to breath deeply.

I settled into my new room on the eighth floor at Duke University Medical Center and contemplated my situation. It was March 2008, and I had just had a double lung transplant. It was the first time that it really came home to me that I had another person's lungs in my chest that were allowing me to breathe. It was the first of many times that I thought about the donor and his or her family. I could scarcely imagine the pain and suffering they had just gone through.

I needed to be stable enough to be allowed to go home, but at the same time, needed to rely on the skill of the doctors and nurses to get myself healthy enough to be able to cope without their support. As one of the nurses said, my goal was to get rid of as many of the tubes and support equipment that were attached to me as soon as possible before I was allowed to leave.

My pre-operative canvassing of various fellow transplant patients at the Center for Living, the rehabilitation center at Duke, told me a stay in hospital of between ten days and two weeks was likely after the transplant. Being the goal-oriented person that I am, I set my sights on a target of a ten-day hospital stay.

I counted eight tubes that were coming out of my chest and side. Most were drainage tubes, where dark fluid flowed into transparent plastic measurement boxes that sat at my bedside. An epidural wire came from my back and extended into a primitive looking box that slowly dispensed the pain-killing drugs that kept me comfortable. Every thirty minutes or so, I would blow into a box-like device that measured the volume of my breathing, as well as exercised the new lungs.

Prior to the surgery, I had no idea if the operation would leave me in pain or not. Some of my Center for Living colleagues, or "classmates", had commented that it was the most pain they had ever experienced, while others said that it was more uncomfortable than painful. Personally, at the moment, I was in no discomfort, other than the fact that I had always thought that epidurals were for pregnant ladies, not for a young guy like me.

The incision on my chest was covered with a single strip of tape. I could feel the crude-looking staples (probably a hundred or so) that kept the incision together. The scar itself was probably around 24 inches long, and ran from armpit to armpit across my chest in a clam-like shape. I would cough up mucus and other such stuff from the depths of my new lungs from time to time, and the nurses had helpfully provided a special red cushion, shaped like a heart, to hold against the chest incision during such episodes of coughing. No one actually said that it was to prevent the chest cavity from bursting open during an impromptu coughing spasm, but that is what it seemed for, so I used it assiduously each time I felt a cough coming on.

I was propped up in the bed in a sitting position. Although it was the best position during the day, I found that it was very difficult to sleep upright.

The days were filled by doctors and nurses coming in and out of my room – checking, checking, and re-checking my vital signs. The day typically started at 4:30 a.m. when a phlebotomist – a different one every day, it seemed – would come waltzing into my room to draw my arterial blood.

Another phlebotomist would come around the same time to draw blood from a vein for the various daily lab tests that they performed to ensure that all the indicators were heading the right way. The blood from the vein was not an issue, as the blood could be taken from an intra-venal site that had already been established. No big deal. The arterial blood, or the blood gases as they were known, was a different matter.

The phlebotomist had to drive a razor sharp knife into the artery at the underside of my wrist to get the sample of fresh arterial blood. Often, he would make a good incision first time, and the torture would be over in seconds. Sometimes, it was not quite so easy. The first jab would miss the artery, and the phlebotomist would dig around a little more until he struck the artery. The pain was excruciating and I had to steel myself every morning not to shout out in agony. I smiled to myself at the irony of not feeling so much pain at the transplant surgery, only to be punished by the relatively minor procedure of a blood test. And to add insult to injury, it always took place around 4:30 a.m.

The nurses would buzz in and out of my room after that doing their checking and counter-checking until the surgeon, Dr. Davies, arrived at around 7:30 a.m. As he strode into my room every morning in the hospital, he was surrounded by a gaggle of obsequious minions, who seemed to cower at his every word. It amazed me how the six or so medical doctors that accompanied the surgeon on his morning rounds could be so intimidated by him. He would not waste his valuable time on trivial things, such as "good morning", but would go straight into asking specific questions and looking for very quick answers from his team.

He would barely look at me, the patient, as his eyes roamed over the dials and indicators that were clustered around the room. For him, the most important thing was there was no sign of infection from the surgery and that the delicately balanced immuno-suppressant drugs were doing their job in ensuring that my body was not rejecting the precious new lungs. The next most important thing to him was that the patient was walking.

That was not an issue for me, as I was a determined walker who was regularly seen walking at my snail's pace round and round the pulmonary unit. The staff had mapped out the one-eighth of a mile route on the institutionally gray walls of the unit, and I proudly recorded each step on a chart in my room.

"Is he walking?" Dr. Davies would curtly ask his staff. He seemed to relax when he was told that, yes, I was indeed walking. One morning, I overheard him remonstrating with a patient in the room next door. His voice was raised as he was obviously irritated by reports that this patient was not walking at all.

"If you don't walk, you are going to waste the lungs you've got. Should I have given them to someone else?" This was enough. I saw the patient out of bed and shuffling around the corridor, walking circuits of the floor moments later.

After sixty seconds or so of his presence, Davies would typically swing around and stride out of the room, certainly without a "good-bye" or a "have a good day". He was a busy guy. The sigh of relief that the nurses in the room let out was tangible once Davies and his entourage left the room to continue their rounds. Nevertheless, despite his lack of bedside manner, I will be forever grateful to Dr. Davis for his surgical skill that saved my life.

Next came my morning chest x-rays. I was collected by a grinning orderly in a hospital uniform, who would sit me down in a wheel chair, load up all my boxes and drips and push me through the hospital to the x-ray unit, where I had my daily dose of radiation.

As I was not allowed to eat or drink anything, and my only nutrition came from my glucose drip, I was losing a significant amount of weight during my hospital stay. Consequently, whenever I left my hospital room, I would start to shake with cold from being so thin. I would always ask for a blanket to keep me warm during these early morning spins along the corridors.

After the x-rays, I was returned to my room. I could hear breakfast being served to other patients in the pulmonary unit, but as I was not allowed anything to eat or drink due to the risk of aspiration into the lungs, there was no breakfast for me. People often complain about the quality of hospital food, but I never did. To me, it looked and smelled delicious, mainly because none of it passed my lips.

Rise and Shine – It's Bronchoscopy Time!

Then around 9:00 a.m. I could hear the light trundling of the dreaded bronchoscopy cart. I would hear it coming down the corridor long before I could see it. A smiling Pedro would put his head around the door and say: "Good morning! Are you ready for your bronch?"

He always came with a burly orderly who would carefully spray and wipe down the three foot long scope with a kind of quiet relish. It wasn't always clear to me what the orderly's role was, apart from spraying down the scope. Maybe he would actually hold down the patient if he decided to struggle much during the scoping procedure, I wryly speculated. I decided not to find out, and just lay back and let the process happen.

As the tube goes down your nose, you cannot help wondering if there is any other equally unpleasant medical experiences that you have to suffer. I'm sure there are, but the bronchoscopy experience must be a leading candidate. The whole process lasts about five minutes, but it seems a lot longer! I have never been mugged, but at the end of the examination, when the tube is withdrawn, you are left feeling beaten up. But each day, through each procedure, and as I relished each breath I took, I knew that I was getting closer to my goal of leading a normal life.

Julie and her dad, Larry, would usually be at the hospital early in the morning to keep me company and to find out what was going on. Usually, they would be in the room by the time the surgeon, Davies, would make his appearance. But the bronchoscopy experience was too much even for them. They would look at each other and say "Coffee?" They would nod at each other. Yes, time to go down to the hospital cafeteria. That would take about 20 minutes, so they would miss the entire ordeal. Lucky them.

CHAPTER 9

Better and Stronger

My stay in hospital passed slowly: Saturday, Sunday, Monday, Tuesday, Wednesday, Thursday. Each day I spoke to Alex and Riley on the phone and they never failed to buoy up my spirits with their cheerful banter. The doctors were pleased with my progress, as the various tubes were being removed and my overall accessory pile was getting smaller and smaller. The doctors were talking openly that perhaps I could get out the next Monday, which would be exactly my target of ten days. I was taking regular walks around the triangular floor where my room was, and charting the distance on the wall of my room. Eighteen laps of the corridors made up one mile.

At the beginning of the week, I needed a nurse, or Julie or Larry, to come with me during my walks. I was slowly getting better at walking, my breathing was clearer, and I was more adept at guiding the two stands-on-wheels that held all my boxes. I had asked Julie to bring my running shoes so I could walk in comfort without using the dreadful hospital slippers. The nurses and doctors who came into my room were always amused that I used to lie on my bed in my hospital gown and running shoes. They knew I was a real marathon runner.

There is a certain bonding that takes place among lung transplant recipients as they are going through a rough, life-or-death experience. Although each patient is different, there are more commonalities than differences, which creates a strong bond. So it was with my friend Jeff, who, as I described previously, had received a lung transplant about three weeks before me. He was characteristically smiling, and his mere presence lifted my spirits. I had met Jeff a week or so prior to my receiving the call. He was already back at the Center for Living for his post-surgery rehabilitation while I was still on oxygen, waiting for the call. He came to visit me several times while I was in the hospital and the fact that I could observe his progressive return to health and mobility helped me through the often painful tedium of my hospital stay.

Although drainage tubes were being removed from my chest, I had to have one additional tube inserted into my stomach, a common procedure at Duke following transplant. The doctors were waiting until a few days after the transplant surgery for me to recover some strength before inserting the stomach feeding tube, called a percutaneous endoscopic gastrostomy (PEG) tube.

I was wheeled down to the surgical ward early on Thursday morning, a week after my transplant. Under a mild sedation, the doctors quickly, efficiently and painlessly inserted a tube into my stomach, some six inches above my belly button.

As I was partially awake, I could talk to the nurse who was at my side during the procedure. I have always found that I talk a lot more when I am nervous. I remember saying to the nurse – maybe slightly overdramatically – that survival was nine-tenths mental attitude, which was what I had heard from a survival expert on the Discovery Channel. The nurse agreed with me and said that I had a great attitude. I lay back and felt the pressure sensation on my stomach as the feeding tube was put in place. At least I would be able to eat something now, albeit only liquids, and all through the stomach tube.

There is a lot of time to think when you are in the hospital, especially at night, when you are propped up in bed and cannot sleep. I made a mental list of the things I wanted to do when I got back to full health. I needed something physically challenging that would help in my recovery. How about a triathlon?

A triathlon is a multi-sport endurance event consisting of swimming, cycling, and running in immediate succession over various distances. Triathletes compete for fastest overall course completion time, including timed "transitions" between the individual swim, bike and run components. It is physically grueling event, which can only be completed by the fittest and most determined of athletes.

The "standard" triathlon is the Olympic distance of a 0.9 mile swim, a twenty-five mile cycle and a six mile run. Slightly shorter is the fastest growing and most popular triathlon event in the United States, termed the "sprint" distance, which consists of a 750 meter swim (a 400 meter swim is common in pool-based events), a twelve mile cycle and a three mile run. The master event of all triathlons is the "Ironman", conceived in 1977 by a group of individuals with undoubted sado-masochistic tendencies, consisting of a 2.4 mile swim, a 112 mile bike ride a 26.2 mile run, all in one day.

I decided to break myself in gently and to start with a manageable triathlon once I was ready: the sprint event. Poked, prodded and tethered as I was to what seemed like a million monitors and tubes, it was a grandiose thing to plan for, all the more so considering that a mere few weeks before, I could barely walk to the mailbox. But for me, it marked a return to life and health that just a few weeks before had seemed to be hopelessly slipping away.

Breathe and Let Go

One of the preparatory talks we received pre-transplant was from a double lung transplant recipient, Tiffany Christensen, who is also the author of the book "Sick Girl Speaks". Tiffany had not only received one new set of lungs in 2000, but she also received a second set in 2002 when her first new set were rejected by her body. She had suffered from cystic fibrosis since the age of six months and was enduring all the challenges of lung transplant again with her new lungs.

Based on her extensive experience with doctors, nurses and medical facilities, she was well qualified to make some pithy observations. One comment in particular resonated with me. She said that the way she coped with such vast medical attention through her young life was that she "gave in" to the process as opposed to fighting it. By giving in, she certainly didn't mean giving up on her will to live or her desire to beat her illnesses. By giving in, she meant surrendering to the relentless process of medical care, doctors' visits, treatments, blood draws, x-rays and all the rest of the steps in her ongoing care. She had made a conscious effort to stop trying to analyze the situation and to go with the flow of her treatments. She had mentally handed herself over to her medical team and let the process take over. In short, she decided to let go of all the "stuff" that was not going to help her with her recovery, and to focus her full attention on becoming well again. She recognized that the "letting go" was an extremely important part of her healing.

As for myself, a goal-oriented Scotsman whose idea of a good time is to run a twenty-six mile marathon under four hours, it was – and continues to be – a challenge to just "breathe and let go." But there has been so much about my situation over which I had no control, that I have little choice but to go with the flow myself, and I have always found it helpful to keep Tiffany's words in mind.

******

I had not been given any information about the donor, except for the fact that the lungs had been helicoptered in to Duke. I had read that some organ recipients feel guilty that they had received another person's organs. I felt many emotions while I lay there awake, but guilt was not one of them. It seemed to me that the death of my donor was entirely independent of my need for new lungs. I did wonder often about the donor family, and the pain they must be going through. I just happened to have the matching criteria of being the right size and having the same blood type as the deceased person. Of course, I felt enormous gratitude at the courageous decision of the donor's family to donate the organs of their loved one. I did not know how I was going to express my gratitude to them. I would have to think about it. I drifted back into a light sleep.

Step Forward, Step Back

By Friday morning, one week after my transplant surgery, two of the largest chest tubes were ready to be removed, one from my left side and one from my right. The fluid that was coming out of the tubes was now yellow, not the bleeding red of earlier in the week. Two young doctors came into my room and confidently announced that they were going to remove the two remaining main chest tubes. I was asked to lean over to one side and take some deep breaths.

On a specific command, I felt a sharp tug on my right side as the doctors deftly pulled out the plastic drainage tube. I stifled a cry, as it really pulled on my raw flesh as the tube came out, but seconds later, the doctors were applying a dressing on the open wound, and taping it down. I breathed a sign of relief. The worst seemed to have passed.

I settled down in my bed for the next hour or so, with Julie and Larry keeping my spirits up. I did not feel bad, just a little beaten up and tired. However, as time went on, I started to feel light headed. My nurse who regularly checked my blood pressure noticed that it was a little low. She did not seem unduly concerned, and said she would keep an eye on it.

Some time later, a doctor came into my room to check on the patched up wound from which the right side chest tube had been extracted. She asked me to roll over onto my left side so she could gain access to the dressing. Even from my twisted vantage point, I could see her eyes widen in alarm. I could see that the dressing and the sheets around me were soaked red in blood. She rushed from the room, and returned with a colleague, and the two of them reapplied the dressing to stem the flow of blood.

The nurse scuttled back into the room and took my blood pressure again. It was going down. I felt very light headed and lay back in my bed. Moments later, the other lung transplant surgeon, Dr. Lin, strode into the room, and took control. He came round to my head and said, "Gavin, can you hear me?" in a raised voice. I could hear him perfectly well, but I could barely respond, as I felt so weak.

"Put the tube back in," he barked at the two attending doctors who were hovering nearby. That was one of the most unpleasant experiences I had during the lung transplant process: the re-insertion of a chest tube into a raw flesh hole in my right side. I breathed in and out exactly as the doctors instructed me, but the pain was excruciating as the tube slipped back in.

I was losing blood through a ruptured blood vessel in the right side of my chest. The nurses rushed to get blood to give me an emergency blood transfusion. It was the only time in the whole process that I was really scared that I was about to die. I could only think about Julie, Alex and Riley, and all the fun that we had had over the years.

Julie and Larry told me later that as soon as the surgeon walked in, they made a hasty exit, as the room was far too crowded with doctors and nurses all flapping around me. The noise drowned out the beep-beep of the monitors around my bed, which were replaced with shouted orders, the bright lights and the general chaos.

After the blood transfusion, the surgeon, Dr. Lin, came back into the room to talk to me. He was Asian, and a much friendlier version of Dr. Davies. I was glad he was there, as his confidence reassured me that I was going to be alright.

He explained that he was almost sure that I had had a ruptured blood vessel that had been kept closed by the chest tube that was in my right side. The removal of the tube had opened the blood vessel, which had caused the intense bleeding. He explained that the only option was to surgically open up my chest again and go in to tie off the ruptured blood vessel. He said that he would perform the surgery the first thing the next morning.

Up to that point, I knew I had had a relatively easy ride as far as lung transplants go. Some bumps in the road were almost inevitable, we had been warned, and this was my one. Julie told me later that seeing me back on oxygen really made her afraid, as it seemed that I had gone from being oxygen-free just after the transplant surgery to being back on the oxygen again. It seemed I had just taken a big step backwards.

I had a telephone conversation with my mum in the late evening. She was staying in Denver along with Julie's mother, looking after Alex and Riley. She gave me some confidence, saying that the surgeons really knew what they were doing. She assured me that I would do fine, and I drifted off into an uneasy sleep.

I had a restless night, as the nurses performed another blood transfusion before I went to sleep at around 10:00 p.m. Julie spent the night in the hospital room with me, curled up uncomfortably in a chair next to my bed. The nurses told me that they had transfused about four liters of blood into my body. Given that the average human body contains about five-and-a-half-liters, it reflected how dangerous the situation had been.

The next morning, I had my blood gases taken, and usual blood draws, but no x-ray. The cheerful orderly came to collect me around 7:00 a.m., expertly transferred me to a bed on wheels, and wheeled me down to the operating room.

Before I knew what was happening, I was back in the post-operating recovery room, slowly coming out of the anesthetic. A surgeon who I had not met before came to see me. He didn't spend long with me, but he said that the procedure had gone well, and that as soon as they had opened up the right side of my chest again, they could see the leaking blood vessel. They had tied a knot in it (yes, really, that's what he said!) and that it should be fine now. He said it was vitally important that I used my blowing device that exercised my lungs. "Use it every thirty minutes for the next twelve hours," he advised.

Back in my room, I clung to the blowing device like it was a life preserver. I used it every ten minutes for the rest of the day, until I could puff on it no longer. I resisted falling asleep until late into the night so I could use it over and over again. This time, I knew I was going to be fine.

CHAPTER 10

Discharge

By the Monday morning of my stay at Duke Hospital, I was feeling much better. During the morning audience, Davies had said that I could go home the next day, Tuesday. I felt elated. I knew that I had been really well taken care of at Duke, but I was anxious to get out of there and get back to the hotel that we had called home for the past two months.

My next challenge was to get to grips with the feeding tube routine and my daily medications regime. I hadn't been paying as close attention to the nurses as I should have been as they administered my medicines at specific times of the day.

The feeding came first. Two or three cans of nutritious but artificial liquid food were poured into a transparent bag on a stand at the bedside. A little pump pushed the liquid through the narrow tube that was connected to my stomach tube. I was surprised that there was absolutely no sensation as the liquid slowly flowed into my stomach. Obviously, there was no taste sensation, as the food was going straight to my stomach, but neither did I get any sensation of 'fullness' once the feeding was complete.

The medicines came next. I knew from the pre-operation briefings that medications and discipline were going to become a big part of my life. Up to the point of my discharge from the hospital, all the medications and insulin had been administered by the nurses.

I had temporarily become a diabetic due to the high dosages of methylprednisolone, an anti-inflammatory drug, which had been given to me during the transplant surgery. It was time I learned, with Julie's help, how to do it for myself. I had a sheet of the medications, and an order was placed at the local Walgreens pharmacy for the mountain of prescriptions.

As one of the biggest fears of any organ transplant recipient is rejection of the organ by the body, the most important medicine is the anti-rejection medicine that suppresses the body's natural immune system. I took, and still take, three anti-rejection medicines every day: Prograf®, Immuran® and prednisone.

Prograf is probably the most critical to get right, and weekly blood draws are taken to measure that the level of Prograf is being maintained. Prograf is a twice daily regime, taken at 9:30 a.m. and 9:30 p.m., each and every day, without fail. I counted up that I would take eight separate prescriptions every day, and two over-the-counter supplements.

To keep the medicines organized, I had a pill box that had twenty-eight compartments organized into seven rows and four columns. This box would ensure that they did not get mixed up and that I knew which ones to take at which time of the day. I could not miss a single dose, so had to ensure that I refilled prescriptions several days before they ran out.

It is still amazing to me that the transplant pulmonologists and transplant coordinators have the skill and knowledge to be able to prescribe medicines in such exact quantities and to read the blood work reports like a pilot reads an airplane's control panel.

A Brief History

Lung transplantation is a relatively young procedure. The first transplant of a complex and embedded organ was the kidney in Boston in 1954, so kidneys have a good thirty year start on lungs. James Hardy of the University of Mississippi performed the first human lung transplant in 1963, but the patient only survived for 18 days. The first successful single lung transplant was performed by Joel Cooper in Toronto, Canada, in 1983, with the first successful double lung transplant performed at the same hospital by the same surgeon in 1986. The lungs were the last of the major solid organs to be transplanted, so pulmonologists are still learning about how to improve success rates among patients.

"Lungs have always been "the bad stepchild" of organ transplants — harder to get, harder to transplant, more prone to rejection and complications than other organs", says Dr.

Scott Palmer, the medical director of Duke University's lung transplant program. Lung transplants were not consistently successful until the mid-1980's, lagging far behind those of kidneys, livers and hearts. And unlike kidneys or liver, which may be transplanted from a living donor, lungs can only be transplanted from a cadaveric donor (i.e. after death). Lung transplants make up only six percent of all organ transplants.

But I am extremely grateful that there is twenty years of experience with lung transplantation; it doesn't sound like much but, without it, I would not be writing this today. Each time I hear about someone who is twelve to fifteen years out from their transplant, I realize how much they are pushing the limits of medical knowledge and experience, and I am thrilled to be one of the people benefitting from their success.

Free To Go

On discharge from the hospital on Tuesday morning – eleven days after I had been admitted (just one day off from my goal of ten days) – we headed back to the hotel, with a trip via the pharmacy to load up on the medications. I still had some six weeks ahead of me in rehab, but I was delighted to be outside. It was what I can only describe as a delicious feeling to leave the confines of the hospital and breathe in the fresh air outside. Just the simple act of breathing in the air and smelling the pine wood smell of some nearby bushes made me feel wonderfully cheerful and optimistic.

As I had come to realize, there were many more people involved in my transplant than just myself. As well as my family and I, there was the hard working and specialized medical team at Duke Hospital, and the donor hospital medical team, but also the donor family. I have a duty, an obligation, to them to ensure that I cherish my new lungs and to make the most of the priceless gift I had been given. I am determined not to let anyone down.

Dr. Davies' parting words to me on the morning of my discharge were "Look after those lungs!"

"Yes, I will." I assured him, but he had already disappeared.

Life of a Transplant Patient

It is obvious to me now that I have to take at least eight daily medications for the rest of my life. This was repeated over and over again throughout my time at the Center for Living and during my hospital stay.

I am still surprised at how often friends will ask me now, "So how long do you have to take your medications?" Often, people believe there is a certain period of time that has to pass before my body gets used to its new organ and the immune system relaxes.

No, unfortunately, that's not how it works. Your body never gets used to the fact that you have an intruder in your chest. Sometimes, it is almost comical to be asked the question. Even my primary care physician in Colorado, whom I consulted on a non-lung issue asked, when he saw my list of daily drugs, "So, are you still taking all these medications?"

My immune system is undoubtedly weakened, but I have found that I can cope with it by taking basic precautions, such as regular hand washing, staying away from people who are sick, getting plenty of rest, along with a good diet and regular exercise. Colds tend to last longer and be more severe than they would be for people with a normal immune system.

Like all the other organ recipients, I will have to take the medications, day in, day out, for the rest of my life. There's no break. Each morning, I load up a small four-compartment pill box with the medicines I need for the day, and carry it around in my pocket. My cell phone's alarm rings at 9:30 a.m. to remind me about the morning Prograf, and I just remember to take the twelve o'clock, five o'clock and 9:30 p.m. dosages. That's just the way it goes, and while the regimen can be tiring, each time I see the white caps of the array of prescription bottles, I know that they are doing a fine job by keeping me alive.

We returned to our hotel that we called home while we were staying in North Carolina, near Duke University Medical Center. The first few nights were difficult, as I was still reeling from the impact of the two surgeries, the influence of the swath of drugs that I was taking, and the fact that I had slept very badly while I was in the hospital. Day and night had merged together, and I found that I was not tired at night, but exhausted during the day. It took quite a few days for my body clock to adjust.

Julie took the fact that I was immuno-compromised very seriously, and spent a full day cleaning and disinfecting the hotel room – cleaning everything from the walls to the phone receivers – to protect me from lurking bacteria. Since then, we continue to be very careful about taking precautions such as hand washing and staying away from sick people, but we have a more realistic view of what is acceptable.

There is always a tinge of trepidation at being discharged from the hospital, as you no longer have the assurance of dedicated medical staff to help answer any questions, or reassure you that you are doing things correctly. I still count my lucky stars that Julie has a background in medicine and pharmaceuticals so could help me navigate through the maze of medical terminology and prescriptions.

I took all the medications in liquid form while I was in hospital, as I had so many intravenous entry points into my body. Now I was not longer in hospital, I had to take the pills orally. Because I was not allowed to eat or drink anything by mouth, apart from the medications (I got all my nutrition through the infamous tube in my stomach), I had been instructed to take a small amount of specially prepared "thick liquid" that I ingested through the corner of my mouth, not the easiest of processes. The thick orange-juice flavored liquid protected my lungs from any damage that could be caused by ingesting liquids of normal consistency, like water.

One of the areas that caused me the most anxiety was the fact that I had become a diabetic since the transplant, due to the high dosages of powerful anti-inflammatory drugs that I had taken. That meant a routine of stabbing my fingers, measuring my blood sugar levels and injecting insulin. I had no experience of diabetes, as I did not have it before the transplant and did not know anyone who had it. Once I understood the management regime that I faced, I developed a huge respect for diabetes sufferers who have to deal with the intensive routine every day of their lives. In my case, I was only a diabetic for three months, until my body could regulate the level of insulin in my body again, after the intensity of the operation.

But while the diabetes lasted, that was where my father-in-law, Larry, came to my rescue. As a former railroad telecommunications specialist, Larry had virtually no medical knowledge or expertise. Nevertheless, once he knew that I was on the list for transplant, he got on an airplane and flew from Tucson in Arizona to North Carolina to be with Julie and me (Julie's mom, Henna, and my mum, May, were already in Denver, looking after Alex and Riley). Larry helped Julie and me immeasurably over the weeks leading up to the operation and while I was in the hospital, acting as a steady, level-headed influence during the turbulence.

After I was discharged from the hospital, he took charge of the box of diabetes equipment and set to work. At 6:00 a.m. every morning, he would come into my room while I was only half-awake, say, "Morning, Gav," take my hand, rub down one of the fingers with a sterile wipe, and stick me with the lancet. After reading the meter for my blood sugar level, he would retrieve the insulin from the fridge, measure out the right dosage and cheerfully stick the syringe into my arm. At the various times during the day, he would repeat the procedure to ensure that my insulin levels were right. I don't think I could have coped with this additional requirement without his help. He even extended his nurse's training to at-home intravenous drips and became adept at taking blood pressure measurements twice daily.

The Center For Living

One of the most cherished beliefs of the doctors at Duke University Medical Center was the value of exercise and activity as an essential component to the healing process. The Center for Living was the central platform of that belief.

The Center for Living is a large gymnasium-type building on the fringes of the Duke campus, hidden away in a leafy suburb of the main hospital buildings. There is a running track around the interior of the building, with exercise equipment and an exercise floor in the middle of the running track. When patients first arrive at Duke for an evaluation, they are told how important the Center for Living is in their recovery process. Then they are signed up to begin their exercise program regardless of their current state of fitness. Many transplant patients are overweight, and are firmly informed that they need to slim down before their operation. The day prior to my discharge from the hospital, Dr. Davies told me that I was expected to show up at the Center for Living the very next day. I knew the lung transplant patients like me were scheduled for the afternoon slot, from 12:30 p.m. to 4:30 p.m. (the mornings were reserved for heart transplant patients), and were expected to finish a six week course of at least four days a week. The session was split into four distinct exercise blocks, all closely supervised by a team of enthusiastic respiratory therapists. The day after my discharge, I reported for duty at 12:30 p.m. sharp, dressed in my habitual running shoes, track suit pants and sweatshirt.

I had lost a lot of weight again while I was in hospital, and my legs felt like matchsticks. Under normal circumstances, exercise is my favorite pastime. I had always considered myself to be the fittest person I knew. But today, standing at the exercise machines, waiting my turn for the leg press to push out 20 pounds, I felt unbelievably weak. Obviously, we were not allowed to do any arm exercises due to the proximity of the lung surgery, but we were allowed, even expected, to do the routine of leg exercises. I finished as many exercises as I could and decided that I felt even worse. As our small group moved over to the floor exercises space, I spoke to one of the respiratory therapists.

"I'm feeling sick. I'm not sure if I can do any more." It was, after all, the day after I had been discharged from hospital.

"Not to worry," she said, cheerfully. "Here is something to be sick into. Just keep it beside you!" as she held up a waste paper bin and handed it to me.

I finished the session, walking slowly around the running track, and biking on the stationary bicycle, but by 4:30 p.m., I was done for. I was glad to see Julie's smiling face there to pick me up.

After the first session back at the Center for Living, the daily routines gradually became easier as my body got stronger. It was incredibly satisfying to make my way, however slowly, around the track under my own steam, without towing a steel oxygen tank. Nevertheless, when I got to the end of the first week, I was relieved to have the weekend to rest before attacking the track again.

CHAPTER 11

Rehabilitation

My rehabilitation program at the Center for Living went on for six weeks after my transplant. I did not mind the regime, involving light weights, floor exercises, stationary biking and walking. I believed that exercise was the key to health and vitality, and I had always enjoyed exercising, even under these conditions.

I exercised every day, except Tuesdays, when I went to the Duke clinic for lab tests, which took up most of the day. I would get a chest x-ray, blood drawn for analysis, and pulmonary function tests.

The pulmonary function tests were one of the most important parts of the assessment. By blowing into a tube with all your might, the doctors could assess how the lungs were doing. The results of the tests measured the speed of the breath coming out of your lungs in the first second (known as FEV_1) and the amount of air that was being pushed through your lungs in the first second (known as FVC). The FEV_1 measure was probably the most valuable predictor of how the lungs were doing.

In the years before my transplant, I would dread doing pulmonary function tests. My breathing had been pathetic and I knew it. As a former competitive swimmer, I knew well the satisfying sensation of taking in large gulps of air, and exhaling a lungful of air in a single smooth movement. Prior to my lung transplant, I could barely take in a breath without coughing, and my exhale was feeble. I knew the sensation of a strong exhale, and that wasn't it.

When I first consulted a pulmonologist in 2004, my lung capacity had been around the sixty percent level of predicted, not good, but not critically poor. By 2007, due to my lung disease, my lung capacity had shrunk to around thirty percent of predicted, which was much worse. No wonder I was having trouble doing the slightest exercise; in fact, it was a wonder that I was functioning at all.

Now, post lung transplant, my pulmonary function tests showed a lung capacity of sixty percent again, and it rose every week by a couple of percentage points, as my tolerance of exercise improved. I now looked forward to the pulmonary function tests, eagerly anticipating a lung capacity increase.

In addition to the lab tests and pulmonary function tests, I would have an appointment with one of the pulmonologists. I usually saw Dr. Steele. He would look at my lab results, listen to my breathing and tap on my back. Generally, he was pleased with my progress and the health of my lungs. I was always relieved when the consultation would only last around ten minutes, which meant that he felt comfortable enough with my progress to not spend any more time with me than necessary.

Jeff was a good friend during the weeks of rehabilitation at the Center for Living. We would measure our progress against each other, although I knew that he was having a tougher time that I had due to his earlier complications. His positive attitude never wavered though, as we counted through the various exercises that were set out for us.

We used to laugh when we had the floor exercises, with various light weights and stretchy elastic bands, as we would invariably fall asleep for a few minutes while lying on the floor. We would wake up with a start when the instructor announced a new position. The fatigue was part of the recovery process from the surgery, but it made us laugh. It was one of the few times during that period that I found humor in my situation.

Stomach Wrap

As the weeks passed, I felt stronger and stronger. However, I was aware that I had one more surgical hurdle to clear. As part of Duke's medical treatment protocol, they recommended that each lung transplant patient receives a so-called "stomach wrap" if there is any evidence of gastroesophageal reflux disease (commonly known as GERD), or acid reflux disease, which is defined as chronic symptoms produced by an abnormal reflux in the esophagus.

As far as I could tell, most lung recipients, myself included, suffer from some level of acid reflux, which is dangerous, as it means that stomach acid can be aspirated back up through the esophagus and into the lungs, causing what is known as Aspiration Pneumonia. To combat this condition, the surgeons perform a stomach wrap or

Nissen fundoplication, a surgical procedure to treat gastroesophageal reflux disease.

In a Nissen fundoplication, the upper part of the stomach is wrapped around the inferior part of the esophagus and stitched into place. This reinforces the closing function of the lower esophageal sphincter, so whenever the stomach contracts, it also closes off the esophagus instead of squeezing stomach acids into it. This prevents the reflux of gastric acid back up the esophagus, and potentially into the lungs.

I was scheduled to go back into the hospital to get the stomach wrap in the following four weeks. The idea did not fill me with eager anticipation, but I knew it was another necessary step on the road to recovery.

Another issue that always concerns the doctors is rejection. Your body's immune system protects you from foreign invaders such as bacteria and viruses. White blood cells called lymphocytes detect the foreign invaders and signal your immune system to attack them. Transplanted lungs are made up exclusively of "foreign" cells, so your immune system, which cannot tell the difference between good invaders (the transplanted lungs) and bad invaders (like bacteria and viruses), will try to attack and destroy them.

To help to reduce such attacks, the transplanted lungs are matched for blood and tissue type prior to the transplant. However, even with a good match, the body's immune system thinks that the new organ is a foreign invader and attacks it.

Rejection occurs when your immune system attacks your new lungs. Immuno-suppressant drugs are prescribed to "slow down" your immune system. But even with the anti-rejection medications, we were told that it is common for transplant recipients to have at least one episode of rejection. Rejection is most common during the first few months following the transplant surgery, but it can occur at any time. Small bouts of rejection were not worrisome and could be handled if treated immediately, but it was the more severe and chronic rejection that was the most serious.

In the months following my transplant, I had three episodes of rejection. After a scheduled bronchoscopy, I would get a call from Cindy, my lung transplant coordinator, who would let me know. My heart would sink when I heard the news. The very word 'rejection' is enough to send a shiver down my spine. However, although it is scary, rejection does not mean that the new lungs have failed, as a mild rejection episode can be reversed with medications, and my three episodes were treated successfully. It is just a constant reminder that you cannot take your new lungs for granted – ever.

Focus On What You Can Control

As I rested in the hotel in the mornings, and exercised at the Center for Living in the afternoons, walking around the track or pedaling on the stationary bike, I had time to contemplate where I was and the progress I had made since the lung transplant. One thing that was ever-present in my mind was the drug regime I had to follow as a result of my transplant. It seemed overwhelming to me. What if I forgot a dose? What if I got the dose wrong and took too much or too little? What if...? An event came to mind that helped me immeasurably to limit my concerns to areas that I could control, as opposed to those that I could not.

A few years ago, I was on a flight scheduled to land at a busy Washington DC airport. As the airplane approached its destination, the pilot announced that, due to air traffic control delays, he was instructed to adopt a holding pattern until a slot became available for us to land. He said there could be a delay of a half-hour or so. This came on top of a late departure, which meant that the scheduled arrival time was about two hours later than expected.

My heart sank. I was going to be really late. I was going to miss my connecting flight, which would probably mean an overnight stay in DC. I would miss a meeting I was scheduled to attend, and that wasn't good. I started to get agitated.

"You alright?" The lady in the seat next to me looked concerned.

"Yes, I guess so, but I'm going to be really late, and we are in this holding pattern, and the flight is already late, and I'm going to be really late, and…" I wasn't making much sense. I could feel myself starting to sweat. Then she asked me one of the most profound questions I have ever heard.

"Can you influence the fight?" she said, quietly.

"Pardon?"

"Can you influence the flight?" she repeated. "Can you make us land any sooner? Can you make up the time that has been lost?"

"No, I can't," I replied, thinking that it was rather obvious.

"Well, why are you worrying then? If you can't influence it, then why waste your energy worrying about it?"

It struck me how many things there are to worry about for lung recipients. I knew how lung transplant recipients experience much higher rates of acute rejection than all other transplanted solid organs, and that how cancer is one of the complications of chronic immuno-suppression. Ah great, more things for me to worry about.

In a recent edition of a newsletter targeted at lung recipients and their families, a contributor had written about how she would avoid Walmart and Target during 'flu season, presumably to avoid the risks of catching something unpleasant. Another contributor wrote about how "I realize that sooner or later I will have to deal with a kidney transplant and/or dialysis." Something else to worry about. A friend recently emailed me and asked: Don't you lie awake at night and worry that something may become "unplugged" from your new lungs while you are sleeping?" I said, no, I hadn't thought about it before, but, yes, I could start worrying about it now she mentioned it.

At my last routine visit to my transplant physician, he mentioned that we needed to be mindful of (i.e. start worrying about) things like my propensity towards developing cancer (statistics tell us that twelve per cent of us develop cancer within the first five years, which incidentally, means that eighty-eight percent of us are cancer-free). Over fifty percent of cancers are skin cancer, not to mention the effect on my kidneys of my twice-daily Prograf. Great, more things to worry about.

That evening, I mentally tallied up the shopping list of things I had to worry about since my lung transplant: my weakened immune system makes me more susceptible to catching colds and 'flu, the drugs are damaging my kidneys, I could develop skin cancer, I now have high blood pressure and high cholesterol, so I could have a stroke, and probably a few others I could not remember. Yikes, quite a list! Worrying is pretty much a full time job.

Then I had a realization. What if I followed the advice of the lady on the airplane a few years ago? What if I only occupied myself with things I could control, and limited my worry to them, and them alone? What if I did not worry about the things that are out of my control?

Areas like medication compliance are worth worrying about, as they are within my control. My regimen of taking medications at 7:30 a.m., 9:30 a.m., 12:00 p.m., 5:00 p.m. and 9:30 p.m. is entirely my own responsibility, so I should make sure that I comply with it. Measures like lathering up with sunscreen or drinking lots of water with my medications are also within my control, so I should worry if I am not doing those things.

But, as for what statistically might happen, I don't have control over many areas, so I needed to let them go. But someone has to worry about them, right – the immuno-suppression, the high blood pressure, the cancer risk, and all the rest? Okay, so let my physician worry about them. He is highly trained, highly intelligent and it is his job to worry about his patients. Why not pass all the things that are available for worry on to him? That way, I won't be burdened with things I cannot control and over which I have no influence.

Ever since I have adopted the "no worry" approach, I have felt much more upbeat and optimistic about this whole transplant thing. Sure, I still worry about the things I have control over, but I leave the worrying about all the other "what ifs" to my physician and his brilliant team. I believe I should focus on what you can influence, not what you can't. In short, I have learned to enjoy and appreciate every day, take a deep breath and let go – of the anxiety, the stress and the things I cannot control.

Back to the flight into Washington DC several years ago: I didn't miss my connection, I didn't miss my meeting, and everything turned out just fine.

CHAPTER 12

Going Home

I had the stomach wrap surgery in mid-May of 2008. Compared to the lung transplant, the stomach surgery was easy. It only required a four-day hospital stay.

When I woke up from the anesthetic, my stomach was quite bruised and I felt as if I had been punched several times. The surgery had been laparoscopic, so there were several – I counted six – small puncture wounds where the surgeon had gone into my stomach to perform the wrap. But again, compared to the lung transplant, the stomach surgery was not a big deal.

I was still 'eating' through the feeding tube in my stomach. I was very much anticipating completing the stomach-wrap surgery and getting the go-ahead from the surgeon to start eating proper food. As I lay in bed, I felt good enough to be discharged but, despite several requests to the surgeon each morning he passed by on his rounds, he stuck to the schedule of keeping me in for four days after the surgery.

On my discharge from hospital, I was allowed to take 'clear liquids' by mouth for two weeks. That meant water and chicken broth, but little else. The strange thing was that I did not feel particularly hungry, as I had not taken any food or drink by mouth since the night before my transplant, some two months before. So I kept to the nightly regime of filling up my feeding bag at 6:00 p.m. and letting it run, with its whirring little motor, until 8:00 a.m. the next morning.

Technically, I was taking in enough calories through the feeding tube to keep me fuelled up, but in reality, it was not enough to allow me to put back on some of the weight that I had lost. I weighed myself every morning, but my weight seemed to stay constant. After the two weeks passed, I progressed to 'dark' liquids, so at least I could enjoy a black coffee to help pass the time. You do not realize – until you can't do it – just how much time you spend on food: shopping for it, preparing it, and eating it. That space gives you a lot of time to think. I used the time to appreciate how lucky I was to have reached this far. At long last, "going home" was on the near horizon for me. I agreed with Dr. Steele that I had one more clinic visit before I could go back to Colorado. His preference was that I stayed under his care for at least the first year, returning every month or so for a clinic visit. I readily agreed. I couldn't imagine, after everything I had gone through, entrusting my care to anyone else.

To say I was very pleased to be on a one-way flight back to Denver to be home in time for my daughter Riley's seventh birthday was an understatement. This was a celebration that the physicians had said that I would not see without a transplant. I wondered what they would want to do with me once I was back, and if they had matured as a result of their exposure to this event in their lives.

Although I was ecstatic to be going home, I was also a little nervous to be so far away from my medical experts at Duke. However, I also knew I would have to sever the umbilical cord at some point, and that I could do so just three months after my transplant was a terrific achievement. To be on the safe side, I wore a surgical mask during the flight.

I had been away from home for four months. When I left, I had been tethered to the oxygen concentrator in the middle of the house, and oxygen tubes ran throughout the house so I could move around. Now, I was breathing on my own, and felt great because of it. Julie had already sent the oxygen concentrator machine back to the oxygen company, along with the piles of portable oxygen tanks that had been stacked in the garage.

I guess I thought that once I got back home, everything would be fine. But my body was still adjusting to the onslaught of medications. I felt more tired than usual, and I was still thin. I still used the feeding tube at night to get my nutrition until I got the green light from the physicians to start on solid foods.

Once I got the go ahead, I had to eat with care. Due to the stomach wrap, the tube through which food flowed to get to my stomach was severely restricted. I had to chew much more thoroughly than before to ensure that the pieces of food were small enough to pass through to my stomach. If I ate too fast, I could feel the food backing up in my esophagus and had to stop eating to allow time for the food to flow again. The stomach issue continues, which forces me to eat more slowly, chew food well and appreciate food more.

I was overjoyed to see Alex and Riley again. Although they had flown out twice in the past four months to visit Julie and me in North Carolina, I had not seen them for the past six weeks. It had never wavered from their minds that I would come back from North Carolina "fixed" from lung disease. Riley in particular was delighted that I no longer had the tubes on my face to breathe. She quietly confided in me the first evening I was back: "I didn't like the tubes, Daddy."

Looking Back

On one of the quiet evenings after I was back home, Julie and I had a chance to decompress and reflect on the events of the past few months. We were alone, with no visitors, and the kids were in bed.

"What was the worst moment for you over the past few months?"

"There were quite a few 'worst' moments, it's hard to think of one specifically," she said. "Definitely when you were told that you were going to have a lung transplant was bad. Everything seemed so up-in-the-air, so uncertain. No one seemed sure what to do. Also, seeing you get thinner and thinner, and having a harder and harder time to breath was difficult for all of us. And waiting while you were on the waiting list was not easy either. Lots of uncertainty. Would the lungs be the right ones? Would they be a good match? Would your body accept them? I jumped every time the phone rang!"

What were the best times for you?

"I remember the relief I felt when you came out of surgery. I was bracing myself for the operation to last ten to twelve hours, as Davies had said. Then I actually saw Davies walking out to the elevator five or six hours after you had gone into surgery. I remember thinking "What's he doing out here so soon? I almost went over to him to ask him. Your surgery was easier than they had expected, which I am sure has led to your quick recovery.

"I also enjoyed meeting you from your rehabilitation sessions at the Center for Living after the surgery. I could actually see your recovery taking place, see you getting stronger and stronger, day to day, as you exercised there."

How did it feel to have your husband so sick?

"It was awful. I knew that there was a possibility that you were going to die, but how do you have a conversation about that? We explained everything to Alex and Riley. We all knew what one of the outcomes could be. We did our best to stay positive, the stay upbeat, and to hope for the best. There were many stories about how successful lung transplant could be, so I trusted that the hospital we had chosen was the right one at the right time."

Navigating the Maze

The process of going through a lung transplant is like navigating your way through a thick and jagged maze. Quite apart from the medical challenges – am I strong enough to get through the trauma of surgery, would a donor be found in time, would the lungs fit? – there are organizational challenges that can be overwhelming.

My experiences led me ask the question: how could the system be improved to make it more penetrable to ordinary folks? Not easily is the answer. What would happen if you did not have access to the internet? Or if you could not speak to specialist physicians informally for advice? Hospitals operate in a competitive environment, so it is hardly in their interest to make it easy for potential patients to compare apples with apples when looking at published performance. And the insurance companies? They probably do not want to encourage easy access to transparent information to allow their insured customers to make more informed choices at an increased cost. The system is deep and complex. The medical challenges are only part of the battle.

Before getting to Duke University Medical Center, Julie and I had to find our way through the many stages that required all our determination and tenacity. The following are just some of the tasks we were faced with:

- Once we realized that I was being turned down by the University of Colorado Hospital, we had to get on the internet and start searching for alternative hospitals. The University provided no help in guiding us towards alternative lung transplant programs;

- Each hospital's website is different, so it required quite a lot of searching, especially as we were looking for a program specializing in high risk cases. We read about each program, had to note down the contact details, and call them;
- Each call required more digging to get to the right person, who invariably would not be available, so they would have to return the call;
- Once we got to speak to the right person, we would have to explain what we needed. The most common question was: why were you turned down by the University of Colorado Hospital? Detailed explanations were needed. Many hospital turned us down flat at that point ("If the University of Colorado Hospital can't help you, then I doubt that we can either.");
- We had to request a letter from the transplant physician at the University of Colorado Hospital regarding my medical issues. That in itself took several phone and reminder calls;
- We had to request twenty-two copies of all my medical records from the University of Colorado's medical records department, which required several visits in person to persuade the clerk that the copies were needed the next day (not two weeks from next Tuesday). They copied the scans onto compact disks, but would not copy the paper results, so we had to go to the copy shop to replicate the inch-thick stack twenty-two times;
- We had to figure out from our insurance company which hospitals would accept our medical insurance and provide them with detailed explanations as to why we were looking for out-of-area hospitals for treatment;
- We had to confirm with each hospital that they would indeed accept our medical insurance, which required us talking to a finance officer (often not the most customer-friendly of individuals). In fact, one of the hospitals, the University of Pittsburgh Medical Center, which did not accept our insurance, helpfully offered to assess my case with an advance of $500,000 in cleared funds;

- We had to bundle up twenty-two FedEx packages with the medical records, address the packages to the right person at each hospital, and send them out;
- Follow-up phone calls were required to request an appointment for a work up, and to confirm that the right person had received the packages, and that they were being placed in front of the right decision-maker at each hospital;
- We conducted telephone interviews, whenever possible, with members of the surgical teams to assess their comfort and experience with high risk cases;
- Post-operative expenses were reasonably covered, but not pre-operative expenses. Despite having excellent health insurance that covered the cost of the operation, we had to pay the cost of our hotel accommodation ourselves up to the surgery.
- Julie and I own and operate our own consultancy business. The flexibility of being self-employed allowed us to take the time off that the transplant demanded while our capable staff continued to run the business in our absence. The situation would be very different without an understanding employer.

All of these steps were in the context of a patient being on twenty-four-hour-a-day oxygen, and facing imminent death through a progressive lung disease. The sense of urgency was intense, and the whole process tiring and stressful. In my opinion, it would be a vast improvement if hospitals were more willing to share information with their patients about the quality of care in institutions other than their own. Patients should feel they are in a cooperative rather than an adversarial system. For example, if a particular hospital has physicians who are renowned for handling complex cases, patients should be provided with that information. Despite the competitive environment for healthcare services, openness with patients should be a priority to ensure the ultimate goal of all hospitals and physicians: patient wellbeing.

I was lucky in many ways in my ordeal. I had a wife who has worked in medicine and pharmaceuticals for many years, which gave her an ability to effectively communicate with doctors, nurses, pharmacists and other medical people. She personally knew several prominent pulmonologists who were familiar with which transplant centers would be willing to handle more complicated cases. She could help me steer my way through the turbulent waters that are modern day medical insurance and all its intricacies. I had a support group of my father-in-law, mother-in-law and mother, who helped us immeasurably through the most difficult times. I can only be thankful for all their help. I can only imagine how daunting and frightening – not to mention life-threatening – the process would be to a person without the benefit of such support.

Keeping Up The Momentum

Continuing the exercise regime was the key to my recovery. It was recommended to walk one to two miles five days a week, along with other arm and shoulder exercises. I used the local park where I could choose from circuits of one, two or three miles and make sure that I completed my regimen every day.

As the weeks passed, I could walk further and further, as I felt myself getting stronger. Once I got my stomach feeding tube removed in August, I progressed to going to the local swimming pool, where I initially started swimming two, four and six lengths at a time. Within two months of starting to swim, I could cover thirty-two lengths, or half a mile, without getting too out of breath. It was the feeling I had waited so long for: the sensation of my lungs expanding and contracting with the exertion of exercise and drawing in cool clear air, without coughing or spluttering. It was magical.

My walking had progressed to a slow jog, as I had rediscovered my running shoes and starting going at a faster pace. Our dog, Joe, was very pleased when I started to jog again and I delighted in the simplicity of running with my old panting friend.

It was around that time that I definitively decided to shoot for a triathlon early in the following year. From my monthly check-ups at Duke, I knew that my lung function was increasing each visit. It was now around eighty-five percent of predicted, although I could tell that it was improving when I ran or swam.

By December, I could jog comfortably, and I could feel the muscle mass coming back to my arms and legs. I decided to aim for a sprint triathlon in the spring. The looming event was enough to keep me motivated to train all through the winter months, rain, snow or shine.

As the event approached in April, I had a clinic visit at Duke Hospital at the end of March. I was elated to find that my pulmonary function tests were at an all time high at ninety-eight percent of predicted. I had shaken off the mild episode of rejection that was detected in December. I had been training six days a week for the past few months, but I still didn't feel in optimal shape. Ever since the transplant, I had felt tired, more tired than usual, especially when I finished exercising. But I kept going, knowing that the exercise was the best thing for my lungs. Julie, Alex and Riley were very supportive in my training, not to mention Joe, our Labrador, who delighted in the daily romps in the park. I found that the running was the hardest of the three disciplines. I could feel the stiffness in my legs when I began to run, and it felt like I was barely moving compared to how I used to run. Nevertheless, I was determined not to give in.

I completed the triathlon in April 2009. It was a typical Colorado spring day – a beautiful clear sky in a cool temperature. How did I fare? I held my own in the swimming part of the event – 400 meters at full speed – but was a little slower in the twelve mile cycling part – probably my weakest event - and crept past the finish line at the end of my three mile run. I got a great reception from friends who had turned out to watch me complete this milestone event. It felt great, even though, effectively, as the only lung transplant recipient in the event, I was in a competitive category all on my own!

My next challenge is to stay fit and healthy for a long time to come. One question that I have been asked several times by well-meaning friends is "Will your new lungs last for the rest of your life"? That's a hard question to answer. Of course, the logical answer is, "yes, they will last for the rest of my life (because if they fail, that would be the end of my life)."

But what they really mean with the question is "will your lungs give you a 'normal' lifespan (in the seventy-five to eighty year range). My usual answer is that I don't know, but my goal is to be a long-term survivor.

The statistics on lung transplant survival are quite sobering. At the Duke University Medical Center, the one year survival rate is eighty-one percent, and the three year survival rate is seventy-six percent (slightly better than the national average three year survival rate for lung transplant of sixty-seven percent).[1] However, these numbers have to be viewed in the context of the median age of lung transplant patients and any other medical conditions.

I have established contact with several other 'long-term' lung transplant patients who are twelve to fifteen years out from their transplants. Given the youth of the whole concept of lung transplant – only twenty-three years of experience – logic suggests that survival rates will only rise in the years to come. It makes me feel immensely special – as if I have been singled out for survival – to receive a new set of lungs that have saved my life. I feel that I am gaining immense benefit from those who have come before me, the real pioneers in the science and art of lung transplant.

Diagnosis?

So what was the lung disease that brought my life to such a grinding halt and necessitated a lung transplant?

I was diagnosed in 2004 by doctors at National Jewish Health as having idiopathic pleuroparenchymal fibroelastosis (shortened to IPPFE). As far as I can determine, this disease is very rare and little is known about it. One of my physicians at National Jewish Health, Kevin Brown, MD, co-authored an article that was published in Chest[2] (the official publication of the American College of Chest Physicians) in 2004. This article described the phenomenon of IPPFE, but said that it had only ever been detected in five (yes, five) patients. The number seems excruciatingly small. How could anyone draw any substantive conclusions from such a small sample?

Even after my old lungs were taken out of my chest for the transplant, and the pathologists could examine them in

[1] Source: Scientific Registry of Transplant Recipients; www.ustransplant.org
[2] Full reference: Chest 2004 Dec; 126(6): 2007-13

detail, they were none the wiser about the intricacies of the disease, such as how I got it or how it could be treated. All they could tell was that it was very efficient at shutting down my lungs.

I have wryly thought many times that I was pretty unlucky to have contracted such a rare condition – if there are approximately five billion people in the world, and five people have got the condition, my chances of contracting it were one in five billion. At those odds, I should be buying lottery tickets!

In the months before my transplant, I was desperate for help from any source, living or otherwise. There were times when I would hear or read something about the complications of lung transplant, which would make me upset, or I would be cheered up by some positive story of survival and success. These are familiar highs and lows for anyone suffering from a serious illness. I often heard our experiences as lung transplant patients being referred to as an emotional roller coaster, and I believe it. But the question I asked myself, and still mull over, is where does God or religion fit in?

I found myself doing a good deal of praying, especially as I lay awake at night in bed breathing through my oxygen tube. Most evenings, Julie, Alex and Riley would lie on our bed and we would hold hands and say The Lord's Prayer. I had grown up in an educational environment where religious ceremonies were shared in school, guided by the Church of Scotland, a Presbyterian church shaped by the Scottish Reformation of the 1560s.

As I had never been to North Carolina before my trip to Duke, I was not aware of the deeply religious sentiment in the southern states of the United States. It was quickly evident, through the number of people I saw reading bibles in the various waiting rooms of the hospital clinic, that the religious penetration was much greater than I was used to. A usual good-bye after you met someone was "God bless you," and people often said, when it was evident (usually by the oxygen tubes) that you were not well, "I'll be praying for you." I received a 'prayer shawl' from a Catholic church group, I was on a

Unitarians' prayer list, and a Farsi friend ensured that I was being prayed for at a mosque in Tehran.

I was humbled and grateful for this support, as it meant I was being helped by friends far and wide. At the same time, I must confess that I always felt slightly ill-at-ease, as I could not reconcile my own health and well-being to that of my donor and God's role in delivering a new pair of lungs.

The central question to me was this: by praying for my health and survival when I needed a lung transplant, what was that saying to my unknown donor? They deserved to live as much as I did. Would God indulge in a system of merit – someone might die so that someone else might live - or was God not involved at all? If God wasn't involved, what was the point of praying to God to be allowed to live? Still, I am happy to accept any help from whichever quarter it came. In the end, I have decided to be happy that I have survived and thrived regardless of any spiritual circumstances that led up to my transplant and beyond. I have made the conscious decision to accept it, to breathe and let go, and to acknowledge that that is enough.

CHAPTER 13

Donors and Recipients

One of the unique features of whole process of lung transplantation - or any organ transplantation for that matter - is that more people are involved than just the patient and his or her family.

When I first understood that I needed a lung transplant, several of my non-medical friends asked a question such as "When are you going to have the operation?" They did not understand that organ transplants are not scheduled like other surgical procedures. There is no bank of organs that the surgeons select from, like there is with, say, blood donations.

There is another party to the process: the donor family. Without the selfless generosity of the donor families, who make the courageous decision to donate their loved ones' organs in the most difficult circumstances imaginable, there would be no organ transplantation. As an organ recipient, I feel an enormous debt of gratitude towards my donor and his or her family.

Due to medical privacy considerations, an organ recipient does not get any information about the donor. I don't know his or her age, sex, origin or background. All I know is that he or she had the same blood type as me, and that he or she was roughly the same size (five feet, nine inches) with the same size of chest cavity so the lungs would fit. I received my lungs during a weekend that was spring break for high school and college students, so I imagine that I have the lungs of a young person, but I really don't know.

Julie, Alex, Riley and myself wrote thank you letters to the donor family about five months after the transplant, which were passed on to the hospital for forwarding. It is the donor family's choice whether they want to be in contact. I have not received any information from them, although I continue to hope that they will get in touch with me when they are ready. If they don't, I hope that they will find solace in knowing that their generosity saved my life. Here is the letter I wrote to them on the anniversary of my transplant.

March 11th, 2009

Dear Donor Family,

I wanted to write you another letter as we approach the first anniversary of the passing of your loved one. I received both lungs of your loved one on March 14th, 2008.

I am very conscious that without your kind agreement to donate the organ, I would not be writing this letter to you today. Your donation has allowed me to get the lung transplant that I needed to save my life, so that I have been able to spend the last 12 months in better and better health with my wife and young family (Julie, Alex, aged 9, and Riley, aged 7).

It is difficult to adequately express my gratitude at receiving the lungs. I understand that it has meant heartbreak for you. I can only hope that you may feel some sense of purpose through knowing that your loss, and your loved one's organs, have done so much to benefit other people. It would mean a lot to me if you feel able to get in touch. I would like to express my gratitude to you either through a letter or in person. If you would like to make contact, please get in touch with your hospital, and they will contact me via my hospital. I hope you feel able to do this.

With very kind regards,

Gavin Maitland

I understand that it may be very painful for the donor family to make contact with the organ recipients. I contacted some other lung transplant recipients to ask them about their experiences, which have been very inspirational. A few of these experiences are set out below.

******

Mary Hardy had a lung transplant at Cleveland Clinic in 2002. After she got home, she wrote a letter of thanks to her unknown donor family. A month or two later, she received a reply from the family of her donor, and after completion of the paperwork, they exchanged letters and telephone calls, and agreed to meet. The donor family said there was something rather unusual that Mary should be aware of before they met: it was the fact that they were Amish.

The summer after the transplant, Mary traveled four hours by car with her two young daughters to Applecreek, Ohio, to meet the family of her Amish donor. She was immediately struck by the simplicity of the community's lifestyle: there were no cars, everyone dressed alike in an old-fashioned style, and there was no electricity. They appeared very different to a conventional community on the outside, but immediately Mary found them to be extremely warm and welcoming on the inside. The community was very family-oriented, with large families and a wide circle of friends. Her donor, a highly respected member of the community, had been forty-nine years old when he was killed in a bicycling accident. He had three brothers and three sisters, and Mary met all of them, and many more members of the community.

Mary was treated like she was the most important person in the world by the Amish – an honored guest warmly taken into this unconventional community. A dinner was held in her honor, with around 100 members of the community present. Mary was only forty years old when she had the lung transplant, the mother of two young daughters, aged four and ten. The Amish community was especially pleased that their tragic loss had allowed a young mother to survive and continue to look after her children.

When the donor, Joseph, known as Junior, had been in the accident that gave him fatal brain injuries, his family said that after the third day of life support in hospital, they felt that his soul had left his body, and they made the decision to end the life support system that was keeping his body alive. When they were approached by the physicians about the possibility of being an organ donor, they said they just knew that that is what Junior would have wanted, so they readily agreed.

Mary considers herself to be blessed, not only at being given a second chance with her new lungs, but also to have been allowed into the special but reserved world of the Amish community. It opened up a whole new avenue of life to her, into a community whose members do not get caught up with the so-called conveniences and gadgetry of modern life, and where there is a tremendous focus on the family and communal life.

Mary has been down to Applecreek about five times in the past seven years, and has spent the weekend there. "As well as for me, it is a wonderful enrichment to my children's lives. I have photographs, taken discretely, of my two daughters playing happily with Amish children," she said. "They are a wonderfully positive influence."

******

Jack Austin received a bilateral lung transplant in 2008 at Shands Hospital in Florida. Despite writing a letter, he has had no contact with his donor family and has no information about the donor.

"I wrote a thank you letter to the donor family just six months after my transplant," he said. "I was a little anxious about writing, as I was seventy-one years old when I had the transplant, and was nervous that the donor family might have wished that the lungs had gone to a younger person. But I will try again, probably at my first transplant anniversary."

******

Dana Siegel had a lung transplant at Methodist Clarian in Indianapolis in 2003. Although she had telephone contact with the mother of her lung donor nine months after the transplant of her left lung, it never progressed to a physical meeting.

"I called the mother of my fourteen-year-old boy donor the day after my husband and I walked our daughter down the aisle to get married. I had just received her information in the mail. I wanted to thank her for me being able to have so much fun planning and attending the wedding. We cried and talked a long time, but she has never contacted me again. I called a few times and left messages, but she has never called back. I send her a card on the anniversary of the transplant."

******

Karen Couture received a bilateral-lung transplant in 1996 at Shands Hospital in Florida. Her donor was an eighteen-year-old man who had been killed in an automobile accident. After her transplant, she wrote letters to her donor family that were sent via the hospital. The months passed, but she did not expect a reply. Two years after her transplant she wrote another letter simply saying that she would like to know a little bit about her donor, but only if and when the family was ready. This time she received a reply directly from the donor family who agreed to make contact with her. As she observes, some families are not ready to make contact with the recipients, and it may take some time until they are ready.

When she got the letter, Karen had to resist the impulse to telephone them right away. Instead, she sat down and composed a letter to the family of the young donor. The letter led to a phone call, and they sent Karen a photograph of Justin, her donor. "It's strange," recalls Karen. "But his picture looked exactly like I had imagined him to look like."

The family invited Karen to come and visit them. They live in Florida's Panhandle, so Karen made the nine hour journey to see them by car. She was very touched by the way the donor family was so welcoming and how they opened their home up to her.

She had expected to visit the family for only a few hours, but ended up staying several days. They visited the grave of their son and paid their respects, which Karen really appreciated. Justin had been killed in an automobile accident while he was selling donuts door-to-door one Saturday morning in 1996. The accident happened on the road that led from their home into town, so the family drives past the site almost every day. The accident site is marked with a small memorial of two baseball bats formed into a cross with a pair of cleats.

Karen has stayed in touch with her donor family over the past eleven years. She sent them the medal she won at the Transplant Games, a biannual celebratory athletic meeting of transplant donors, recipients and their families, and a copy of her book, "The Lung Transplantation Handbook." She also sent them flowers on the anniversary of her transplant, although Karen finds those gifts so insignificant compared to what she has received.

They have got together three or four times since that first meeting, and have become quite close. The father walked Karen halfway down the aisle when she got married in 2006. She gets calls from the father from time to time, as he likes to stay in touch, although she is very respectful of the relationship, as it is one with such unique characteristics. "I feel so grateful to them when we get together," she said. "However, anything I do seems inadequate as they have given me so much."

In this particular case, Justin's parents, Ronnie and Anita Richards, were anxious to make contact with the recipients of the organs of their beloved son. They were curious how the recipients were doing, as they would be carrying a part of Justin. They were very pleased when they received a letter from Karen saying that she would like to meet them. They invited her to a sports tournament in their home town that they had founded in Justin's name.

As Ronnie recalls, as soon as he saw Karen, he knew exactly who she was. He describes how good it felt to hug her and feel her breathe with Justin's lungs. The Richards welcomed Karen into their family at once, and found that she fitted in perfectly, as if they had known each other all their lives. Karen shared Justin's passion for baseball, and was even writing a book about the sport.

As the donor family, Ronnie and Anita are aware that Karen is afraid that she has not done enough to express her thanks to them. "But there's nothing to pay back," says Ronnie. "It was a gift, pure and simple."

Even though it was thirteen years ago, Ronnie and Anita think about their son Justin every day. For Ronnie, every Saturday morning is just like the day Justin had his accident. It was a very difficult decision to donate Justin's organs. Although he was clinically dead, Ronnie and Anita felt that any moment he would open his eyes or reach out his hand to them. Justin had only twenty-four hours on life support before they made the decision to donate his organs.

It seems like there were dozens of questions from the doctors: would they agree to donate Justin's lungs, his heart, his kidneys…? Ronnie felt the questions were like bullets coming at him. He was pleased for the organ recipients, and the benefit they would get from the organs, but also sad for himself at his own loss.

However, meeting Karen and knowing that she had done so well with her new lungs made it all worthwhile. Ronnie feels an enormous amount of gratitude that Karen has used the lungs well.

"She has done us good," he said. "I hope that everyone in our position can reap the rewards of meeting a recipient like Karen.

Meeting the recipient is a blessing for both sides. Karen has been our angel."

******

Each lung transplant recipient has his or her own story. My friend Jeff, who provided me with such inspiration, had a complex journey up to his double lung transplant. His story provides a harrowing example of the obstacles that some patients face – and overcome.

In January 2006, Jeff got the first indication that all was not well. He and his wife, Janeen, had gone for a full day of medical testing at a wellness clinic in Dallas, which included a chest CT scan. The doctor identified what he termed 'broken glass' on the CT scan of Jeff's lungs and also noted that his spirometry tests, which measure the speed and volume of a patients breath, were lower than expected. The doctor looked at Jeff and said, "It's likely you have pulmonary fibrosis. You are in for the challenge of your life."

Although the diagnosis was a shock, it was not entirely unexpected. Jeff's brother, Mark, had already been diagnosed with idiopathic pulmonary fibrosis some years earlier, and Jeff had already lost several close family members to the disease. Jeff knew that something was not right with his own breathing, as he used to run every day for exercise but this activity had become more and more difficult. Jeff contacted the same pulmonologist as his brother had consulted and made an appointment. The pulmonologist was brutally frank.

"You are going to die," he said, apparently without feeling. "You have probably got three to four years left at most." As Jeff left the doctor's office, he remembers walking down a long corridor, unable to believe what he had just been told. He was only forty-four years old. It felt like a death sentence. Thoughts buzzed through his mind, not least of who would look after his family when he was gone.

As part of the diagnostic procedure, Jeff had a lung biopsy in the following weeks, which confirmed his diagnosis. In fact, it was worse than he feared. There were seven categories of severity of pulmonary fibrosis: Jeff's diagnosis was the seventh category, the worst one.

He remained with this same pulmonologist for the following six months, but with growing distaste. He felt the pulmonologist had mentally written him off as a hopeless case, so Jeff decided to take matters back into his own hands and look for help elsewhere. He had come to the realization that his only hope for recovery was to get a lung transplant, so he contacted pulmonary specialists in Dallas, San Antonio and Cleveland. As he describes, he felt quite good at this point, despite coughing four to five hundred times a day and suffering three bouts of pneumonia.

"I felt like suffocating in slow motion," he recalls.

His new pulmonologist, recommended to Jeff by his family general practitioner, mentioned that only a specialist institution such as Duke University Medical Center would give him a chance of survival. After a year of research and interviewing physicians at different medical centers, Jeff made an appointment at Duke.

At the same time, Jeff was literally watching his older brother Mark deteriorate. To make matters worse, Mark was additionally diagnosed with lung cancer on top of pulmonary fibrosis. Cancer is one of the conditions that usually rules out a patient for a lung transplant. Although distraught by Mark's serious condition, Jeff and his family were pleased that Jeff did not have cancer.

Then the pulmonologist found a spot on Jeff's left lung. The spot looked like cancer, so he ordered a biopsy of Jeff's lung. The biopsy result returned positive. Jeff had adenocarcinoma, the same type of cancer that was afflicting his brother. Despite this devastating diagnosis, Jeff's doctors proceeded to treat him.

Then, at last, there was some good news. Jeff's cancer was limited to his left lung, and was caught early enough to allow the physicians to be able to at least consider the possibility of a lung transplant. In September 2007, surgeons operated on Jeff and removed the lower left lobe of his lungs. A biopsy following the surgery revealed that the cancer had been eliminated, but that Jeff's lungs were failing fast. As one of the surgeons described it, the lower left lobe was "like an old leather football."

Jeff's next hurdle was to convince the physicians at Duke to continue to treat him. "I want you to learn from me," he told them during a marathon interview session.

"Do as much experimenting on me as you can. I have lost a brother, a mother, an aunt and an uncle to pulmonary fibrosis, so use me for research so you learn something about this disease."

The physicians deliberated for less than twenty-four hours on Jeff's case before they came to the unanimous decision: Yes, they would continue to treat him and get him the lung transplant that would prolong his life.

"But you have a ninety percent chance that the cancer will return in the first year," he was warned by the lead pulmonologist.

Jeff went through all the work up testing in preparation for the lung transplant surgery, which showed that he was in good health, apart from his deteriorating lungs, and that he was cancer-free. He was added to the list on Valentine's Day, and got the call that lungs were available six days later.

The transplant surgery went well and he was out of hospital within eight days. The surgery left him with a few issues, including the loss of half his right diaphragm and one of his vocal cords. He also couldn't cough up any mucus, as he couldn't get his vocal cords to close, so he felt as if he was "drowning in mucus." Some of these conditions required readmission to hospital and additional surgeries.

Jeff endured no less than fourteen surgeries under general anesthetic during his ordeal. As the lead pulmonologists said to him, everything that could have gone wrong went wrong. Despite these obstacles, he continued to walk as soon as he was out of the intensive care unit each time.

"I knew that if I did not walk, I would die," he recalls ruefully. He walked one mile the first day, two miles the second day. He even looked forward to the daily hospital bronchoscopies. One time, the physician who performed the bronchoscopy procedure had to go back in two additional times to clean out all the mucus from Jeff's lungs, but Jeff didn't complain.

"Go back in as often as you need to," he would say cheerfully to the nervous physician. He regarded the bronchoscopies as one of the essential healing steps that he had to go through on the road back to health.

What kept Jeff going through his ordeal? "Well, I have a real strong will and a strong determination," he says. "I don't take no for an answer. I also had a deal with my brother, Mark, that, if necessary, we would allow each other to die with dignity. We would also look after the other one's children if the worst happened."

Has the experience changed him? "I don't waste many hours now. I used to spend time dealing with things that were incredibly unimportant. I don't do that anymore. I have realized that I am not bullet-proof. Also, my appreciation for life has changed. I don't know anyone who has a better outlook on life than I do. I live in the moment and every day is an absolute gift to me."

Jeff's brother Mark passed away in October 2008.

******

During the first few days of staying at the Marriott Residence Inn in Durham, North Carolina, Julie met Agnes, the mother of Tricia, a cystic fibrosis patient who had a life-saving double lung transplant.

As the days progressed, Julie met Agnes at different times, got to know her, and Agnes shared her daughter's story as a lung transplant recipient. Despite my position of being on the waiting list, and despite all I had been through in the past few months, my story paled in comparison to Tricia's.

At the time of meeting Agnes, Tricia was in hospital, waiting for the lung transplant that would save her life. She was in hospital because she was still on a ventilator following the birth, just a month earlier, of a beautiful baby girl called Gwyneth. Gwyneth was delivered by emergency Caesarian-section at a gestation period of only twenty-four weeks. There was no fewer than seventy-five medical staff in the operating room with Tricia for the birth.

Following Gwyneth's premature arrival, Tricia was placed in a medically induced coma for nine days, while Gwyneth faced her own struggle in the neonatal intensive care unit. Tricia was slowly weaned off the paralytic and sedation medications until she was fully awake and aware of everything that had taken place. She remained on a ventilator, which she was to stay on for three months. Less than seven weeks after giving birth, Tricia was listed on the organ transplant list, a rare event, given she was still on a ventilator.

Tricia had a high lung transplant score, but was told that new lungs might be difficult to locate, as her blood type was rare. In the meantime, she walked around the corridors of her hospital unit – where she walked nearly a mile every day – with the help of her ventilator and a walker. She could visit her baby for just a few minutes every day.

On April 2nd, 2008, almost three months after Gwyneth's birth, Tricia got the call she was waiting for from the transplant team that a pair of lungs was available. She endured a nine hour operation as her old sick lungs were replaced with new healthy lungs. In just under three weeks in the hospital, Tricia was discharged to complete her six-week program at the Center for Living.

Gwyneth spent over eighteen weeks in the neonatal intensive care unit. While she remained on several medications to help her premature body grow, she has developed normally without any significant issues.

But Tricia's ordeal was not over yet. Although she did not have any signs of rejection, two months after her transplant, she was diagnosed with post-transplant lymphoma, a form of lung cancer brought on by the transplant. She had no choice but to endure a round of chemotherapy. This first round was unsuccessful in treating the lymphoma, so she was aggressively treated with another four rounds of chemotherapy. By November, six months after her transplant, she was told that the cancer seemed to be in remission.

Tricia had suffered from cystic fibrosis all her life. When she got married to Nate, she was showing more signs that her lung disease was causing her body to deteriorate. With the support of her medical team, Nate and Tricia began trying to get pregnant, realizing that their window of opportunity was extremely narrow.

As the months went by, Tricia's disease had progressed to the point where her doctors advised her to stop trying to conceive and to consider undergoing the evaluation process for a bilateral lung transplant. Tricia went through the week-long evaluation process at Duke University Medical Center to determine if she was a candidate for lung transplant. Fortunately, she was accepted as a candidate, and made arrangements to temporarily move to Durham to be near the hospital.

The day before Tricia was to begin the physical therapy that would prepare her for the transplant list, she found out that she was pregnant. Against the advice of many of her doctors, Nate and Tricia chose to keep the pregnancy despite being told that Tricia and the baby had less than a fifty percent chance of surviving.

As the pregnancy progressed, and as Tricia's health deteriorated, she went into the hospital, which was when Julie met her mother, Agnes. I still hadn't met Tricia when I was discharged from the hospital following my transplant, although it was only a few days later that Tricia got her new lungs. I remember Agnes' jubilant face as she told us the news.

When Tricia was eventually discharged from the hospital, I can recall her determination at the Center for Living as she walked circuits on the track to regain her strength. If anyone ever had the mental toughness to get through a near impossible situation, it was Tricia, her husband Nate and little Gwyneth.

CHAPTER 14

Drivers of Lung Transplant

During the three months I spent in rehabilitation at Duke University's Center for Living, I was exposed to the full spectrum of lung transplant patients; it was a valuable opportunity to share experiences and motivation with the twenty to thirty other recipients who were at various stages of rehabilitation before or after their lung transplants. It also gave me a sense of the kinds of conditions that would necessitate a lung transplant, and where I fell within the range. As it happens, mine was an unusual case: the majority of the other patients were either young men and women who had cystic fibrosis, or older individuals suffering from idiopathic pulmonary fibrosis (IPF) or chronic obstructive pulmonary disease (COPD).

Cystic Fibrosis

Cystic fibrosis is an inherited disease of the secretory glands that mostly affects the lungs, pancreas, liver and intestines. The disease impacts the mucus secretions that protect the linings of these organs. The secretions become thick and sticky, causing mucus buildup, and blocking tubes and ducts, and also increasing the individuals' susceptibility to infections. The disease is passed through the genes from parents to children; people who have cystic fibrosis will have inherited the condition from both parents, who carry the disease but do not have it themselves. The hallmarks of cystic fibrosis are salty tasting skin, normal appetite but poor growth and poor weight gain, excess mucus production, coughing and shortness of breath. Often, symptoms of cystic fibrosis appear in infancy and childhood.

Although it is technically a rare disease, cystic fibrosis is ranked as one of the most widespread life-shortening genetic diseases. According to the Cystic Fibrosis Foundation, average life expectancy is around thirty-seven years old without a transplant. Indeed, the transplant recipients who I met were typically in their late teens or early twenties. These people had suffered their whole lives with breathing difficulties until the disease progressed to the stage of threatening to overwhelm their lungs.

Lung transplant often becomes necessary for people with cystic fibrosis as their lung function and tolerance of exercise declines. Although single lung transplant is possible in other diseases, people with cystic fibrosis must have both lungs replaced because the remaining lung would contain bacteria that could infect the transplanted lung. Lung transplant is considered when lung function nears the point where it threatens survival, usually around twenty to thirty percent. However, there is often a narrow time frame when transplant is feasible as the patient must be healthy enough to endure the surgery.

I was always awed by the cheerfulness with which the "CFers" dealt with the hand that life had dealt them and the determination and strength with which they faced their transplant and recovery. James Watson, for example, suffered from cystic fibrosis all his life which eventually necessitated a double lung transplant to save his life. What is cystic fibrosis really like?

"Basically, any small function made it difficult to breath," he commented. "I always felt that I was behind, no matter how hard I tried. I panted a lot, I would cough a lot, and it felt like I was running in place. Doing any kind of physical exercise made me winded. I was a server in a restaurant, which meant a lot of walking and movement. I would feel exhausted by the end of the shift, and all I wanted to do was to go home to sleep. The coughing especially tired me out."

Post transplant, James is doing extremely well, regularly playing ice hockey and racket ball, in addition to planning his wedding.

Chronic Obstructive Pulmonary Disease

On the other side were recipients in their sixties – not always, but typically from what I saw – who were dealing with one of two main lung diseases: idiopathic pulmonary fibrosis (referred to as IPF) or chronic obstructive pulmonary disease (known as COPD, chronic bronchitis or emphysema). There is no known cause of idiopathic pulmonary fibrosis except that it typically affects people in their sixties and once it is detected there is no known cure, except for a lung transplant.

COPD is different, not in its deadly nature, but that it is caused – in over 90 percent of cases – by smoking. COPD is recognized as a serious global health problem, being highest in countries where cigarette smoking is very common. COPD is the fourth leading cause of death in the world (the three causes above COPD are heart disease, stroke and HIV/AIDS). COPD patients are associated with a high co-morbidity, meaning that they are complex to treat due to other serious health conditions.

Jack Austin was diagnosed with COPD. He says, "COPD, in my experience, is not nearly as bad as some of those other lung conditions, such as cystic fibrosis, idiopathic pulmonary fibrosis, or alpha 1 antitripsyn deficiency. COPD is slow. Unlike them, there is no "you have only two years left" sword hanging over your head.

"I was diagnosed in 1987, but I did not go on full-time oxygen until the end of 2007. You just get progressively shorter and shorter of breath. As COPD progresses slowly, you learn to pace yourself and can continue to be active. I was down to fifteen percent of predicted lung capacity, as measured by my FEV_1 score, but was still playing golf. I would take one practice swing, hit the ball, and then rest a bit before pressing on.

"I am retired, but feel I could have worked at an office job right up to the time I was transplanted. Being short of breath is terrible, but I knew that I could sit quietly and slowly recover. Of course, this activity level was dependent on drugs, especially the inhaled ones. When I received the transplant call, I had to do a nebulizer treatment before I could do the one-and-a-half hour trip to the hospital. I smoked cigarettes for thirty years and I have only myself to blame. Watching others battle cancer and other conditions like idiopathic pulmonary fibrosis, I feel blessed."

A difficult question is posed by medical conditions that are largely self-imposed. Cigarette smoking is largely a choice and people who are suffering from smoking related illnesses – so the argument goes – should not be given priority over people who have become ill through no fault of their own. For lungs, it is smoking. For the liver, it could be alcohol consumption. For the heart, it could be poor choices of diet and exercise. The counter argument runs that smokers, or alcoholics or heart attack victims are living their lives the best way they know how, making changes to improve their condition, and should have access to the same opportunities for medical care as everyone else.

Current medical thinking is that treatment decisions are made on the basis of medical need only, regardless of how an individual acquired the condition. As it would be impossible to accurately assess who was a 'deserving' case or a 'non-deserving' case, priority for treatment on the basis of medical need is really the only way lungs or other organs can be allocated.

CHAPTER 15

Giving Back

In the year following my transplant, I wrestled to find an adequate way to give back in recognition of the gift of life that I had received. It goes without saying that I am very grateful to my donor family, but I want to find a way to appropriately express my gratitude and to make a difference in some way in the transplant community. A thank you letter to the donor family seems so inadequate. There must be more I can do.

One route I have followed has been to help with the efforts of many individuals and organizations to promote the cause of organ donation. This is very important. Mountains of evidence show that the more public awareness that exists about donating organs, the higher the donor rate. Increasing the donor rate is important as statistics clearly show that demand for all types of organs outstrips supply.

In countries like the United States, the waiting lists for organs have grown longer as factors that drive the need for organs increase: populations that live longer, advances in medical science, and medical conditions such as hypertension and obesity (largely responsible for kidney failure). The problem is worsened by a fall in road traffic deaths, which – along with heart failure and stroke – are a big source of the organs that can be transplanted. In 2007, it is estimated that over 7,000 people in the United States died while on the organ donor waiting list. The list currently stands at over 100,000 people, according to UNOS.

The lack of donor organs has given rise to many scandals, particularly in poorer countries, where a black market trade in organs has developed to meet the worldwide need, particularly for kidneys. In India, it used to be legal to sell organs for donation but, after revelations of the exploitation of illiterate peasants, who were often coerced into donating a kidney, the practice has now been proscribed. Chinese officials only admitted as recently as 2005 that its widely reported practice of recovering organs from executed prisoners was true. According to Chinese government statistics, at least one million people in China need organ transplants each year, but only about 10,000 receive them.

A look at the donation rates of several Western countries helps to put the relative rate of organ donation into perspective. In countries like Spain and the United States, the donation rate is more than double that of the United Kingdom.

Country	Cadaveric organ donor rates per 1 million of population; selected countries 2007[3]
Spain	34.3
United States	26.6
France	25.3
Italy	20.9
Ireland	20.2
Canada	14.8
Sweden	14.5
United Kingdom	13.0
Australia	9.0

Given that the number of donors is directly correlated with the number of organ transplant operations that can be carried out, it is worth asking what factors contribute to low donor rates in some developed countries, and whether the rates be increased even further in the higher donation countries.

One factor that plays a role in the low donor rates in some countries is the negative publicity that surfaces occasionally around organ transplant from events that are widely publicized by the media. For example, in 2008, the *Los Angeles Times* reported that four Japanese men with suspected gang ties, who were subsequently banned from entering the United States, received liver transplants at the UCLA Medical Center between 2000 and 2004[4]. The organ recipients also donated $100,000 to UCLA after the operations, which many people found distasteful. Under heavy criticism in the media, the medical center defended itself by saying that it has no mandate to make moral judgments about its patients. Regardless of

[3] Source: Transplant Procurement Management, Barcelona; 2007
[4] Los Angeles Times, "After Livers, Cash to UCLA" May 31st, 2008

its rationalization, the publicity surrounding the transplant was negative and had the potential to discourage potential donors.

The second question is can the rates be increased even further in the higher donation countries? A recent survey[5] has indicated that only fifty-four percent of families are willing to donate a relative's organs and tissue if they are unaware of their loved one's wishes. However, when they know of their loved one's wishes, ninety-four percent say they would honor the request. In the United Kingdom, for example, over two thirds of people say that they would be willing to become donors, but only a quarter have signed the donor registry. In countries like the United Kingdom, and the United States, it has been shown that, when it comes to organ donation, the more publicity the better.

Presumed Consent

Another controversial area is the system of "presumed consent" that is in use in most European countries. Under presumed consent, a person is assumed to be a potential organ donor unless he or she has registered an objection. In the United State and the United Kingdom, the opposite system is in place: potential donors have to opt in (i.e. indicate their willingness to donate their organs on death).

It seems logical that an opt-out system would generate more organ donors than an opt-in system. Look at the statistics for Spain where there is an opt-out system. There are 34.3 donors per million inhabitants, one of the highest donation rates in the world, compared to a lowly 13.0 donors per million inhabitants in the United Kingdom. This seems to make a *prima facie* case for a system of presumed consent.

However, the logic does not always stand up. In the United States, the opt-in system results in the second highest donor rate in the world, at 26.6 donors per million inhabitants. Clearly, there are other factors at work. In Spain, a publicity campaign was run to explain organ transplant to the public and to deflate common myths surrounding transplant. Among the myths: "I am too old to donate my organs"; "If I am a registered organ donor, doctors won't work so hard to save my life"; or "My religion doesn't support organ transplant." All of these beliefs are untrue.

[5] Source: Donor Alliance

The key argument against a 'presumed-consent' system is that it removes a sense of control from the hands of the dying patient and their families. The fact that donation is compulsory might mean that there is more push back from the public around the whole concept of giving a gift of life through organ donation.

It is worth noting that the simple act of stimulating public debate over whether or not to use the system of presumed consent in the United Kingdom raised the number of registered donors by seventeen percent. The key to increasing the supply of organs for transplant seems to be through positive publicity and the resulting increased public awareness.

Increased public awareness of the issues and implications of organ donation is also important, especially when a donor family only has a very short time in which to make a decision. This can be illustrated by the following letter that was published in *The Economist* magazine[6] in response to an article on organ transplantation:

> ***Easing a difficult decision***[7]
> *SIR – I read your article on organ transplants with interest ("The gap between supply and demand", October 11th). I am the father of a seven-year-old boy, Nicholas Green, who was shot and killed in an attempted robbery during a family vacation in Italy. My wife and I donated his organs and corneas to seven very sick Italians, four of them teenagers. We've watched them grow into men and women and, 14 years later, all seven are still alive. Having seen all this I cannot visualize any decision other than the one we made, though to us at the time those people were just statistics on a waiting list.*
>
> *The main obstacle for most people, I suggest, is this: brain death is usually sudden death—a road accident, a stroke, violence—and people arrive at the hospital to find someone they love, who was in good health only a few hours earlier,*

[6] Edition of October 23rd, 2008

[7] Permission to reproduce kindly granted by the author

now dead or dying. Many are too stunned to take it in, others are angry and looking to assign blame; relations between family members may be tense, almost all are confused about organ donation.

To make a major, irrevocable decision there and then in this highly emotional atmosphere, about something they have never thought about before, is just too much for many people. They say no and often regret it for the rest of their lives. On the other hand, of all the hundreds of donor families I have met, I can scarcely remember one who regretted the decision.

If this is correct, the solution is clear: just as with any other important decision, families should discuss the options in calm conditions, when death is still a distant concept. As the overwhelming majority of people in most countries say they would donate a family member's organs if they were faced with the choice, I would expect donation rates to soar.

Reg Green
La Cañada, California

The author convincingly argues that increased public awareness, in particular the discussion of individual's wishes, is the key to increasing organ donation rates.

Getting Involved

Lung problems are often associated with smoking – usually accurately in the case of COPD, but not in the case of cystic fibrosis, pulmonary fibrosis and other insidious lung diseases – so I do not feel that I have a legitimate voice to discourage smoking. I have always been against smoking – as a child I used to hide my grandmother's cigarettes when we stayed with her to prevent her smoking – but I contracted a vicious lung disease. One of my neighbors, a lifelong smoker, told me that she stopped smoking when she learned about my lung disease. She felt ungrateful that she was voluntarily mistreating her lungs when I was having such unprovoked difficulty. But her cessation didn't last long; she was soon back puffing her way through a pack a day, good intentions laid aside.

One path I have followed is to be a member of the Donor Alliance in Colorado. The Donor Alliance is one of fifty-eight not-for-profit organ recovery organizations federally designated by the U.S. Department of Health & Human Services to facilitate the donation and recovery of organs for people who need transplants. The Donor Alliance connects organ transplant recipients with other members of the transplant community, such as patients, health care providers and donor families. The idea is to spread the word as much as possible about the concept of organ transplant. The more people who are aware of organ transplant and its benefits, the better.

At Duke University Medical Center, I also agreed to participate in any medical studies that were requested. As Duke is heavily focused on medical research, I am more than happy to provide any help I can in terms of allowing the researchers to study my progress prior to and beyond my lung transplant.

Finally, I believe that my main obligation is to keep myself as healthy and well, to keep my positive attitude oriented in the right direction and do as much as I can to support the cause of organ donation.

AFTERWORD

I am often asked why I decided to write a book about my lung transplant. I felt I had to write this book for a number of reasons, but one reason in particular was the most compelling. I have always wanted to write a book, and the lung transplant experience gave me a subject that I could really get my head around. I also wanted to give back to the transplant community by writing an accessible account of the lung transplant process that readers could identify with and be more aware of the whole complex and life-saving process. The more people who are aware of the demand for organs and the need to sign up on the donor registry, the better.

But the overriding reason for writing the book came from my ten-year-old son, Alex. I mentioned to my wife that I was thinking of writing a book, and Alex overheard the conversation. He said to me later, "Dad, are you going to write a book?" I replied, yes, I was thinking about it. Without hesitation, Alex replied, "I bet it will be really good!"

Alex's blind confidence inspired me to write the book, as I felt that I could not let him down. His core belief was that nothing could go wrong, and that the book would turn out perfectly. To his mind, why wouldn't it? It was the same positive thought process that he applied to my lung transplant – it never crossed his mind that anything could go wrong, or that there would be anything other than a successful outcome. This is one of the most important lessons I have learned from my lung transplant: a positive outlook and a belief that things will turn out for the best are worth a hundred doctors and hospitals.

Acknowledgements

I would like to thank the many people who helped me enormously before, during, and after my bilateral lung transplant: my beautiful wife, Julie, and children, Alex and Riley, for their faith and fortitude; my dad and mum; my brothers, William and John; my aunts, Ailsa, Dorothy, Kathleen and Margo, for their support from a distance; Julie's parents, Larry and Henna Busboom; Bob Rhoades, PhD; Sidney Braman, MD; Alvar Agustí, MD; the team at Duke University Medical Center, especially Duane Davis, MD, Shu Lin, MD, Mark Steele, MD, David Zaas, MD, and Cindy Lawrence, RN; Tricia Lawrenson, Jeff Drinkard, Jack Austin, Dana Siegel, Mary Hardy and Karen Couture for letting me use their stories; James Richardson; Marc Bozon; our many family and friends who helped out in ways too numerous to mention with phone calls, cards and emails. This network of kind hearts, who assured me that everything would turn out just fine, were an immeasurable source of faith and strength.

And last, but not least, is my donor and his or her family, whoever and wherever you are. A profound thank you from the bottom of my heart.

LaVergne, TN USA
06 January 2010
169015LV00002B/75/P

9 781608 443338